The Little Book on Cancer

by
Dr. Elvis Ali

DR. ELVIS ALI

ISBN:1514283379
ISBN-13:978-1514283370

DISCLAIMER

The information in this book at all times is restricted to education, teaching and training on the subject of natural he alth matters intended for general natural health well-being and do not involve the diagnosing, prognosticating, treatment, or prescribing of remedies for the treatment of any disease, or any licensed or controlled act which may constitute the practice of medicine.
Any questions?
Please email us at:
drelvisali10@hotmail.com

CONTENTS

ACKNOWLEDGMENTS

It is with great pleasure that I acknowledge with thanks...

My entire family in Canada and Trinidad and Tobago who have continued to support and motivate me to educate others about naturopathic medicine. My parents, Hakim, Hazrah, my sisters, Alima, Homaida, Homeeda, Fazida, my children, Hassan, Azeeda, Kareem; nephews, nieces and precious grandchildren, Gursimran, Meheirveer and Shairveer for their encouragement and belief in holistic medicine.

Colleagues in the health care profession: Drs. Ayad, Khoshbin and Michelle, Sam and Yvonne, Ghaznavi, Polymenea, Oh and Wu, Joyce and Frank; Naturopathic Drs. Leo Roy, Yu, Chhoker, Markou and Omar.

Thank you to the colleagues and companies for their assistance in educating the public about preventative medicine: Ecoideas and Biorrific team: James, Rafic, Nathan and Pinder; Canadian Bio, Sangsters, Fion Beauty Supplies Canada, GreenCross Bioceuticals Canada; Wellspings Esthetics and Spa.

My dear friends, Bonita, Pat, Roy, Cindy and Darryl, Janak, Joan, Mei, Lili, Sunnie and Jason, Ellen at *Alive* Magazine, Master Teresa, Jennifer, Ash and Harry, along with many others too numerous to list.

My publisher and editor Sherree Felstead and Lillian Jia who designed the book cover.

AUTHOR'S MESSAGE

Dear Readers,

Recently, naturopathic doctors were recognized by the Regulated Health Provisions Act in Ontario, Canada. This is exciting news, because our industry is under the regulated health professions act that is similar to doctors and other health professions, which means patients are empowered with more choices.

This welcome news validates the information provided in this book. It also balances the knowledge of a medical doctor, Dr. Leo Roy, and myself, a naturopathic doctor.

While studying to become a naturopathic doctor, I had the pleasure of having Dr. Roy as one of my professors. Back then, in 1985, he taught us nutrition and I did my preceptorship in his office on Bloor Street in Toronto before graduating in the very first full-time graduating class in Canada from the Naturopathic College in 1987.

Dr. Roy moved to British Columbia a few years later and I went to visit him. We spoke about the holistic approach to treating patients with cancer. As a medical doctor, Dr. Roy also integrated his medical knowledge with naturopathic medicine, which included various modalities, such as dietary therapy, stress management, supplements and creative visualization to boost one's immune system. Dr. Roy and I decided that it was imperative to make available our knowledge to as many people possible, including our patients, about the disease of cancer. We spoke about collaborating together on writing a book to help educate and empower people, not only on prevention, but also about the importance of boosting their immune system to ensure that cancer doesn't have a chance of invading their bodies.

I was deeply touched that Dr. Roy bequeathed to me his writings before he passed away, so that his knowledge lives on in these pages and in other books that will be published at a later time.

This book combines Dr. Roy's knowledge and experience about the treatment and prevention of cancer, as well as mine.

Thank you for your interest in this book. Whether you are seeking information to prevent cancer or to broaden your options, I hope you will find it very beneficial and empowering.

Sincerely,

Dr. Elvis

A Personal Story:
MY VICTORY OVER LIVER CANCER

My name is Ruth Pericone and I had cancer of the liver. I was given only a few months to live and that was well over 15 years ago! At that time, I phoned Dr. Leo Roy and stated that I had just returned from following treatments at a clinic in Mexico. I had acquired a supply of Laetrile. I needed someone to give me the injections, because my own doctor would not. Would he help me?

"Mrs. Pericone," Dr. Roy said, "I am familiar with Laetrile and its merits. Of course, I will do this for you. However, I have to be frank and tell you that I don't believe it will do you much good."

Upset I replied: "I don't understand. Laetrile is supposed to be a cure for cancer."

"I know it is a remedy for cancer," he answered, "but I cannot accept it as a <u>cure</u>. In years of treating cancer patients, I have never yet encountered one whose condition was not due to a multitude of causes – often as many as 20, 40, 60 or more factors and abnormalities. Single remedies cannot cancel out multiple causes. Causes that are not counteracted will continue to affect your condition. They could counteract your healing, but I don't believe that cancer can ever be totally cured without eradicating all of its causes."

"What you are saying makes sense. Is there anything you can do that can help me?"

"I don't know", he replied. "What kind of cancer do you have?"

"A month ago, my doctors took out half of my liver. Half of it was a solid cancer mass. They sent me home to die, but I am determined I'm not going to die without a fight and without trying everything I can."

"With an attitude like yours, I'm most willing to do everything I can to help," he replied, "but I can't help much by guessing or assuming. Guessing is like playing Russian Roulette with someone's health. That is not fair to you. It can fail; however, there is a way to find answers that might help. It involves learning everything in your life that may have been responsible for bringing on your condition. We can obtain this information by several means. You would have to complete a questionnaire of several thousand questions. I will need all your

medical reports, your laboratory and other tests. I will put all these together with detailed physical examinations and with other tests, which will reveal your body's abilities to heal.

"Healing is done by the liver. Your liver will have little healing power so I need to understand your emotions, your attitudes, the nature of traumas or complexes, your environment, the state of health of every organ of your body and especially the chemicals, poisons, toxins and abnormal substances, which could have starved, damaged and denatured the cells in your liver. We would have to unearth everything that might prevent you from healing. It would be like a detective investigation. With such an amount of information, it is possible to find the major causes of your illness. Once these are known, there are ways and remedies that can offset and eliminate them. If we can correct everything, restore all your healing abilities, it could be possible to overcome your disease. It would be your responsibility to follow all treatments 98 percent perfectly or as close to it as possible. Even with all this, there is still no guarantee of a cure. Only your body knows if it can cure or not. It could take a few months before we know whether you can be helped or not."

This made perfect sense to me.

"When and how do we start?"

Dr. Roy gave me his huge questionnaire, which I answered. I gave him copies of all my hospital laboratory tests, my doctor's findings and reports. We spent hours discussing every angle, digging into every minute problem, deficiency, toxicity, imbalance - anything that might be in disharmony with my individual nature.

I gave him my story from its beginning. I had been upset for years, because I was unable to become pregnant. Tests had revealed nothing seriously wrong with me or my husband. The hormonal patterns and sperm count were adequate. I went on fertility drugs and they didn't work, but still no fertility. We decided to adopt a baby and our application for a child was approved.

Still anxious for a baby of our own, we persisted under a doctor's care. To put my glands at rest, with hopes that they would eventually develop an ability to fertilize, he put me on birth control pills. These produced a blood clot in my lung and I almost died. While in the hospital recuperating, the doctor arranged for a lung scan. The technician misread the doctor's writing and he did a liver scan instead, which showed a tumor in my liver. The doctors promptly scheduled me for surgery and they found a mass about the size of half of my liver. They cut away half of it, sewed me up and sent me home to die. I was unable to accept that I was going to die. Something inside me told me that I hadn't finished my life yet. I had to live. Not just for myself, but for my adopted and loved child.

I was determined he wouldn't be left without having a mother. Every time I looked into his eyes, I knew that I wanted to be alive to see him grow up. In desperation, I kept searching for anything that would help me survive. There had to be a cure for me out there somewhere. I was going to defy my doctors and prove them wrong.

My first visit with Dr. Roy lasted four hours. In short order, he knew more about me than even my mother knew. The massive amount of diagnostic data that came from the questionnaire and my whole life story brought to light many reasons and causes for my cancer. We discussed them and worked together. Everything started to come together in my mind. I realized that there really were possibilities of a cure.

Dr. Roy stressed that therapies cannot be effective as long as I continued to believe that curing cancer was impossible and I continued to live with fears. He would sometime say, "Don't hurry, don't worry, keep joy in your life." I would try repeating these to myself. I used biofeedback tapes to overcome my fears and strengthen my mind.

My fears receded when I visualized myself at an open window and I saw the cancer cells banging at the window and coming straight towards me before I could close the window. With practice, I got to the point where I could close the window before the cancer cells got to me. Eventually, I developed enough strength to mentally see myself throwing fists full of cancer cells out the window and watch them fly over mountains and miles away. There was no more need to close the window of my imagination.

I was given a very strict diet. Dr. Roy prescribed a series of supplements to restore the healing power of my body and to revitalize its immunity and resistance to disease. They consisted of highly concentrated cell extracts of the liver and of other organs for detoxification and elimination. I had to take many enemas to flush the cancer-causing poisons out of my body. There were also herbal remedies. I took a handful of supplements several times a day. Taking all those pills and following such a rigid detoxifying regime was very unappealing; however, I had decided that until God told me there was no more room down here for me, I was going to fight and live.

I was ordered to follow everything right to the letter, or else! I kept in communication with Dr. Roy and I followed the whole program religiously. I read and studied health, reorganized my life to resolve every problem and abnormality. I maintained a positive attitude and morale.

Initially, I felt wonderful. I felt more energetic for the first time in many years. I could feel the supplements taking over, supporting and restoring my organs and life systems, so I took a holiday to the United States with my family. Although I was very thin, I managed to keep up with my husband and child for those two weeks. On the way home, my condition changed. I began to feel really ill. Doctor Roy later explained that when the healing powers come back to life, the body starts to battle all the poisons that had been destroying my liver. Getting rid of them is like getting rid of toxic levels of alcohol during a hangover. One does not have hangovers only from alcohol. We go through this kind of experience when our bodies dump any poison or toxin.

For the following months, I was constantly upset, distressed and miserable and I could not eat. I could feel myself going downhill. I collapsed and took to bed. The treatments produced tremendous pain in my liver and I was nauseous and weak. I was experiencing reactions like I was poisoned and dying. I would wake up in the night and literally crawl to the washroom to take coffee enemas to empty myself of the poisons that were creating my pain, weakness and distress. I would often need several enemas before there was any relief. I experienced strange aches and pains. One of them occurred in an area on my right arm that had been broken years before when I was only six years old. Some aches lasted for a day or two and others disappeared and didn't return.

I seriously wondered if I was going to live, as did those around me. The experience was somewhat like a drug addict struggling to overcome the deadly effects of their drugs. I was 'drying out' from the poisons that caused my cancer. For a long period of time I went through a sort of special hell.

Dr. Roy kept our hopes alive by stating that he did see the pattern of reactions as being that of dying. He thought and hoped that the distresses were those of a body that was engaged in a battle to live. He added that there was no way of knowing how much life force and resistance was left in me to overcome this crisis. If these ran out before my fight was over, I would not make it. If I survived this 'battle', I would have a good chance of beating my cancer.

Not knowing whether I would live or die, my husband and family were frantic. There was nothing they could do, but be patient. Weeks and weeks went by. They continued to surround me with love and encouragement. They cooperated with every effort I made even to the point of changing their own diets, taking the same juices and meals as I did. They began to make changes in their own lives as they saw the changes in me.

Little by little, I experienced change and improvement. The treatments were working! What I had been experiencing is often termed as a 'healing crisis' – a state that many seriously ill patients go through. For the next six months, there were ups and downs. Thank God, mostly ups! I gradually improved.

A year after surgery, I returned to my surgeon. He was amazed that I was still alive. I was still suffering, because I had long bouts of projectile vomiting. He thought there was a blockage in my colon. He assumed this must be from a cancerous tumor. He operated on me again. There was no tumor in my colon, nor was there any tumor in my liver! It had completely regenerated. My colon had been choked by my liver as it enlarged. I bounced back quickly from the surgery and healed fine. Within a week, I was home again. One year later, tests showed my liver to be normal in size and no tumor. Every six months for four years, the same reports.

After four years, I felt better than I had during the years prior to my illness. My energies were strong and my eyes were bluer than they had been in years. Friends thought I was wearing tinted contact lenses. My complexion was good. My skin was soft and wrinkle free – no doubt from the highly nutritious diet that I had been on.

Since the lives of my husband and I had been so fulfilled and enriched by our baby boy, our thoughts turned to adopting another baby. The Christian Adoption Agency was most cooperative. That Christmas, I took home another darling boy. I was deliriously happy and I was again healthy. I had two beautiful children and a wonderful, supportive husband.

That should have been the end of the story, but no. Within a month, I was pregnant! Due to my changed lifestyle and improved eating habits, and in spite of being 38 years old, I went through an easy and pleasant nine months. My delivery was quite quick and relatively easy. Within the next few years, there were two more children – all boys.

My husband Frank and I find our five boys to be a delight and source of pride and fulfillment. They are excelling in their school work, athletic and music achievements. They keep me going in a way I never thought would happen or that I could manage, because I have a fulltime job.

I had been asked by a well-known liver specialist to call him every year and provide him with information about my condition for his records and research. For many years, I was too busy 'living' and forgot to call him. Finally after the birth of my fifth child, I did call. He was flabbergasted that I was still alive, even more so, when I told him that I was now part of a family of seven. To my knowledge, he merely tabulated my success as another statistic of his sterile research.

No notation was ever made that I had followed a different system of managing cancer and a different route to health. Over the years, I encountered doctors, either socially or through appointments for my children and they refused to believe that I had ever had cancer. They were amazed that I had survived cancer. They told me that I looked too well. There must have been a mistake in diagnosis. But my surgeon had all the tumor reports, the tests and the laboratory confirmations. Three hospitals became curious about my case. Their doctors searched through medical literature and they could find no record of a lady who *first was cured of cancer and then gave birth to children afterwards. They concluded I was a medical first.*

Now, in my 50s, I am still going strong and look years younger than my actual age. I owe my life to the philosophy and system that Dr. Roy mastered and the practices presented in this book.

A typical medical comment would be: *"Another case of spontaneous remission."*

The author's comment would be: *"This can be a typical pattern of healing for those with serious and/or terminal cancer..."*

CANCER IS NOT:

- *An evil witch or diabolical sorceress that nonchalantly wanders around seeking innocent victims to destroy*
- *A disease for which we know no causes*
- *A disease for which there are no good answers or cures*
- *A disease only medical doctors know how to treat and control*
- *A disease to fear and dread*
- *A reason to give up on life and living*
- *A tumor*

Cancer does not just happen. Normal healthy cells do not just spontaneously metamorphose into abnormal cells unless they are deprived, debilitated, poisoned and damaged.

Cancer is the sum of all the processes, which transform normal, healthy alive cells into abnormal, damaged, denatured and toxic cells. Tumors are merely the end result of this process. Tumors are *not* the cancer. The process that creates the tumor is the real cancer.

Cancer is a disease of cells and understanding cancer is understanding cells. Treating and curing cancer is treating, normalizing, supporting, sustaining, nourishing, protecting and regenerating cells. The study of cancer is the study of all these points.

Medical research, over generations, has progressively unveiled the secrets of the world inside living cells – secrets that have kept us in ignorance about cancer for centuries. There is no more mystery about cancer; however, there are many complexities. Cancer in each patient is the combination of their body's cells reactions to all the chemicals, drugs, pollutants, radiations that saturate their environment and of all the stresses, hazards and abnormalities of their lifestyles and civilized conditions of living.

INTRODUCTION

To keep the body in good health is a duty...otherwise we shall not be able to keep our mind strong and clear. Lord Buddha

In my private practice I am often asked: *"What can I do to stay healthy?"* And my usual response is: *"There is no one magic pill since our body is so complex and made up of several macro and micro nutrients."* Besides water, we need protein, fats, carbohydrates, vitamins, minerals and trace minerals on a daily basis. Sufficient intake of essential vitamins and minerals is therefore crucial for maintaining overall health and wellbeing – emotionally, physically and psychologically.

I appreciate those who ask me the question, because they are seeking balance in their lives. We are all leading hectic, stressful lives and it is often difficult to maintain balance and experience vibrant health. It is problematic that people are not receiving all the nutrients they need from the foods they eat. On top of that, there are lifestyle excesses, such as alcohol, drugs (antidepressants, antibiotics, for instance), lack of exercise and not enough 'down time' and sleep. Furthermore, as we age, some nutrients are absorbed less efficiently, which requires greater amounts to obtain their benefits. Adding a high-quality formulation of vitamins and minerals that work synergistically with our body type is necessary to experience optimal health.

Antioxidants are also part of the delicate balance. Smog, tobacco smoke and automobile exhaust are just some of the many environmental pollutants that we are exposed to on a daily basis. These harmful substances can build up in the body and form unstable molecules known as free radicals. Free radicals can easily bind with other molecules or atoms, causing chemical reactions in the body. We need free radicals to produce energy and certain substances that the body requires; however, excessive free radical formation can have detrimental effects on our cells and tissues, eventually destroying them. Also, excessive amounts of free radicals in the body have been linked to major chronic diseases, such as cataracts, premature aging, cancer, coronary heart disease and other degenerative diseases.

Certain enzymes in the body act as "free radical scavengers" that neutralize unstable molecules, making them no longer harmful. Besides the body's natural defense, certain vitamins and minerals called antioxidants also help protect it against the formation of free radicals. Many antioxidants can be obtained from foods that we eat, especially fresh fruit and vegetables. However, we now know it is difficult to get enough to fight off the many free radicals generated in our polluted environment.

I will be discussing the importance of dietary needs and supplements more as we move further in the book. What I wanted to emphasize here is how crucial good nutrition and supplementation are as part of the mind, body and spirit equation for the best health, especially when you or someone you know or love has received the diagnosis of cancer.

The human body can be very forgiving. What is required is making a conscious decision to make healthful living a priority.

Cancer is preventable, treatable, conquerable and curable

Believing that cancer is beyond the abilities of science and doctors to understand and master was justifiable during the centuries when we knew little or nothing about cells, their physiology and biochemistry, and the impact that chemicals, drugs and radiations have on them.

We are no longer in the dark ages of science. The era of cancer ignorance is in the past. Libraries of information exist about cells, their nature and functions, how they multiply and divide, and what agents control cell proliferation. It is no longer justifiable to claim that we don't know the nature and causes of cancer.

It is true that we don't know *'the'* cause or *'a'* cause for there is no such thing as a single, simple cause. There are only multiple causes. Cancer is a complex illness. By correlating all facts and causes together, cancer becomes understandable. It is only when we allow our minds to be mesmerized by the misconceptions of past centuries that we have difficulties accepting and mastering the realities of cancer. We need to relook at the whole cancer concept with minds completely free from beliefs and conclusions from the centuries of ignorance and replace them with the scientific discoveries of the last 50 years.

Clear, common sense, realistic awareness of everything about cancer can cancel out our fears and replace them with assurances that there are a multitude of answers available to overcome cancer.

CHAPTER 1:
CANCER IS A DISEASE OF CELLS

Growth for the sake of growth is the ideology of the cancer cell.
Edward Abbey, American Author

When cancer invades the body, it is because of poisons, attackers and abnormalities that transform normal cells into biochemically-distorted, abnormal and sick cells. Now, remember tumors are *not* the cancer. The process that creates the tumors is the real cancer.

Cells are molecular structures of proteins, minerals and trace minerals, oils and thousands of enzymes. Cell nuclei house chromosomes and they govern and control the life, functions, growth and dividing of cells.

Cells are surrounded by, and float in, body fluids like fish in an ocean. In constant contact with all the substances in those body fluids, they are subject to chemical reactions within them. Anyone with high school chemistry knows that it is not possible to place two radically different chemicals in contact with each other without each one reacting with the other. Everything in our body's tissues, organs, fluids and cells are chemicals. They are vulnerable to chemical reactions.

If the inner body's environment (ocean) is healthy, the cells will remain healthy. If the inner body's environment is polluted and full of poisons, the cells will eventually be damaged by those poisons. Nature has created an almost impregnable and formidable protective suit of armor covering the cells: cell membranes – possibly, the most powerful and effective protector of cell structure and function.

As long as the cell membranes are healthy and intact, cells resist all invaders and attackers.

Cell membranes are made up of proteins, oils, minerals and lecithin. They control cell nutrition by selectively allowing the absorption of molecules, which are identical to the original form structure. They repel and reject all substances of nature different to their own special biochemistry, including poisons and carcinogens.

Membranes also play a major role in controlling what cells absorb and control their growth, dividing and multiplying. By powers of a magnetic attraction, cell membranes act as gates whereby needed nutrients enter into the cells.

Deficiencies, denaturing and deterioration of the cell membrane is the start of cell disintegration and its transformation into a cancer cell. It is only when cell membranes succumb to reactions with the toxic chemicals in which they are immersed, and become chemically damaged, that they lose their power to defend themselves and block the infiltrating poisons and carcinogens. They pierce the membrane barrier and enter into the cell organelles, enzymes and other cell components. Cells lose their identity and become cancerous cells. It may take years for body pollutants and poisons to damage, breakdown and destroy cell membranes.

A cell with a damaged membrane, pierced in many places, has its inner structures denatured and destroyed. It no longer functions in normal ways. As cells become over-filled with excesses of any kind, they swell beyond their normal size. When close to double in size, cells will normally divide into two. Their excessive proliferation creates masses of billions of cells. These are tumors.

It is unfortunate that cancer societies and medics constantly spread statements that they do not know the causes and nature of cancer. Yet you will read about them in the media. They are also listed in journals of toxicology. There are no secrets or mysteries. There are keys to understanding cancer. We just have to pay attention.

In all cancers, there are three categories of causes:

- *An inherited predisposing cause* that weakens cells and their resistance to disease.
- *A contributing cause* that overloads all of the body's organs and cells and hinders them from metabolizing toxins and wastes.
- *A triggering cause* such as highly toxic substances that denatures, damages, and transforms normal cells into cancer cells. The most lethal is killing agents known as carcinogens.

Having an awareness about the causes is empowering and the most important step to affect real change. So let us go a little further and look more closely at the causes.

External Factors

The external factors are those that are in our environment, as noted before. Carcinogens are rampant everywhere due to advancements in technology and the pollutants different industries produce.

Environmental Carcinogens:

- Polyvinyl Chloride PVC's
- Polychlorinated biphenyls (PCBs)
- Polycyclic aromatic hydrocarbons (PAH)
- Specific metals: lead, arsenic, cadmium, chromium, nickel, aluminum, zinc
- Minerals when taken in a non-food form, such as supplements
- Chemical fertilizers

Air source carcinogens and radiation:

- Exposure to radiation and radon
- Radioactive potash-type fertilizers
- Radioactive potash fertilizer for tobacco crops
- Cigarettes and secondhand cigarette fumes
- Highly toxic chemical fumes
- Industrial fumes
- Carbon monoxide from road and air traffic fumes
- Fumes from garbage disposal dumps

Pesticide:

- Organo-chlorines
- Organo-phosphates
- Alachlor: the most widely used, primarily on corn
- Captan: used on apples, cherries, grapes, nectarines, peaches, pears and strawberries

- Ethylene-bis-dithiocarbamate: used on potatoes and tomatoes
- Parathion: used on peaches, pecans, walnuts and wheat *(the leading cause of poisoning for workers in California)*

Food-forming Carcinogens:

- The rancid fats from barbecued meats and fishes
- The rancid oils from roasted coffee
- Smoking agents used to smoke foods, meats, fishes
- The rancid, chemically treated hydrogenated oils
- Fried foods, such as chips and fries
- Fast foods
- Hydrolyzed proteins
- Amines + sugars = pralines
- Microwaved foods
- Foods grown in nitrate rich areas

Water- sourced Carcinogens:

- Fluorides, chlorine, chlorides
- Dioxin
- Industrial water-polluting effluence
- Saliva solubilized thallium, used in the mercury for amalgam fillings (Thallium kills instantly on contact)
- Water, wells in nitrate rich areas
- Poisonous soluble of water pipes, plastic bottles and water treatment chemicals

Carcinogenic Food Additives:

- Sucaryl – Saccharin
- Aspartame
- Cyclamates
- Yellow butter
- Nutri-Sweet

- Sweet and Low
- Yellow OB
- Yellow AB
- 1,000 food additives, preservatives, coloring, flavorings

Medical-source Carcinogens:

- The side effects of medical treatments and surgery
- Chemotherapy
- Radiation and radioactive materials
- IUDs and vaginal creams
- Many medical drugs routinely used for chronic ailments
- Diethylstilbestrol and 'the pill'
- Chemical interactions between prescription drugs and the chemicals and drugs in our foods
- Hallucinogenic drugs, Marijuana and Cocaine

Miscellaneous Carcinogens:

- Pyrrolizidine alkaloids
- Safrole and ertragole
- Quinones, phenols
- Ethyl carbonates
- Catechol (catecholamines)
- Vicine and convicine
- Hydrazines
- Glycoalkaloids
- Phenol esters
- Acetylaldehyde
- Canavarine
- Braken fern
- Coumarins
- Cycasin
- Coal tar
- PAH

Internal Factors

Stagnating body wastes from faulty elimination, digestion and metabolism are the internal factors that causes unpleasant and foul-odor gases and bacteria in our bodies, such as:

- Indole
- Hydrogen sulphur
- Methylmercaptan
- Pentamethylenediamine
- Methyguanidine
- Ptomatropine
- Beta-imidazolethylamine
- Indican
- Neurine
- Cadaverine
- Butyric acid
- Muscarine
- Crescols
- Sepsin
- Skatole
- Urobilin
- Putrescine
- Histidine
- Ammonia
- Butoline

Food-forming Contributing Factors:

- Caffeine, coffee, tea, chocolate – methylxanthines: these are chemical cell-damaging agents found in caffeine, (rancid coffee beans or powder) tea, chocolate
- Theobromine, theophylline: constituents of coffee, tea, chocolate
- Alcohol and their additives and agents: acetylaldehyde

- Nitrosamines, PAH: flavoring and coloring agents

Foods that do not provide any benefits to health, resistance, or immunity:

- Fats in meats – pork, bacon, ham
- Scavenger foods
- Rancid wheat germ and ground cereal grains
- Dead foods – denatured
- Canned foods
- Overcooked foods
- All foods prepared with preservatives
- Stale foods
- Dry boxed cereals
- Pasteurized foods – milk, honey
- Chemical imitation – instant, non-foods
- *Coffeemate* and imitation creams
- *Ensure* and similar vitamin and mineral supplements
- Isolated, refined process amino acids
- Table salt

Sugar Foods:

- Soft drinks
- Cakes/pies
- Cookies
- White sugar = glucose, sucrose
- Desserts
- Fruit sugars (fructose)
- Brown sugar
- Milk sugars (lactose)
- Chocolate bars

Contributory Environmental Factors:

- Chemicals in drapes, carpets
- Glues in fabricated woods
- Industrial pollutants and effluence
- High tension wires
- Air Pollutants
- Sprays, pesticides
- Aerosols
- Consumer gases and hydrocarbon fumes
- Industrial fumes
- Cigarette fumes (*Smoking alone is not a sufficient explanation for the occurrence of cancer; however, a combination of life stress and smoking constitute a powerful instigator of the disease.* Eysenck, 1988)

Infections:

- Fungi in the jaw bone
- Cold abscesses
- Root canals
- Viruses
- Mouth and gum infections
- Parasites
- Infected bladder and/or kidneys
- Other abscesses

Chemicals – Drugs:

- Medical and prescription drugs
- Hallucinogenic and 'kick' drugs
- Cosmetics
- Hair dyes

Lifestyle Factors

Dr. Vince DeVita, head of the National Cancer Institute, was interviewed by *Newsweek* in the fall of 1982. He admitted that 80 percent of cancer is related to lifestyle and nutrition, and since that time, over 30 years ago, cancer diagnoses have increased exponentially. We could safely say that stress has been a primary factor, because of the rapid changes we are experiencing in most, if not all facets of our lives.

Our eating habits are erratic and we are relying more on the convenience of readymade, processed and fast foods in which little or no nutrients exist. Ideally, it would be great to receive nutrients from the foods we eat, however, due to the additives, preservatives and chemicals in them, it is unlikely we are getting the vitamins and minerals from our diet. When we include skipping meals, increasing caffeine and alcohol, our bodies eventually become ticking time bombs.

When cancer has been diagnosed, there are general, basic rules about nutrition that every patient must follow. But every cancer patient is a unique individual with needs different from others. Their needs vary according to:

- Age
- Activity levels
- Intensity and tenseness or relaxed, laid-back, slow, low energy, easy-going, slow functioning nervous system, brain and glands
- Metabolism and the body's biochemistry the rate of function
- The nature and duration of nutrient deprivations and deficiencies

CHAPTER 2:
CANCER IS A BATTLE

You never know how strong you are until being strong is the only choice you have. Cayla Mills, Author

No one can live a sheltered life and avoid the cancer-inducing conditions prevalent in the current state of our world. In the presence of carcinogens, our bodies are saturated with additives, preservatives, pollutants and chemicals and they become battlegrounds to keep the disease at bay. Cells struggle constantly to protect themselves against chemical enemies, biochemical deficiencies and imbalances that threaten to destroy them. Unfortunately, those who develop cancer have done little to provide their bodies, minds, emotions and spirit with proper nutrients.

Believe it or not, there is no specific entity called 'cancer'. Cancer cells cannot survive and grow except by feasting on excess pollutants and poisons that saturate the fluids in which they are immersed.

People who have succumbed to the processes that create cancer cells – those whose bodies have lost the ability to neutralize and get rid of all the chemicals, poisons and carcinogens which damage cells - succumbed to the disease, because the cells have been affected by 20 to 60 or more causes. If they are not detected and unveiled, what is not known, of course, assumes the semblance of being a mystery.

Individually, each cause may be simple and not serious in nature; however, the sum total of all of them together becomes a destructive process. Also, the assortment varies with each person. What causes one person's cancer is not likely to be the same combination of causes that destroys the health of another.

Cancer in Comparison with Other Diseases

The body is like a huge jigsaw puzzle with each organ, each tissue and each biochemical functioning as a single component. All diseases are distortions, damages or absences of one or several pieces of the jigsaw.

In minor illnesses, one or several pieces are damaged or missing. In serious diseases there is a larger number of damaged or missing pieces. Those that are damaged or missing have a great impact on the health and normal function of a body.

Here are a few diseases we can compare with cancer:

Colds: Fatigue; exhaustion; lowered resistance; low Vitamin A and C; a high mucus food diet; toxin retention; stagnation; catabolic deficiencies.

Flues: The same as a cold, but more. Toxins of greater toxicity; a much lower resistance; failure of the organs to detoxify; much less Vitamin A and C and deficiency of phospholipids.

Ulcers: Decreased HCl, secretions and digestive enzymes are way too low; an intense, uptight lifestyle – type 'A' personality and serious nature; workaholic; excessive responsibilities; nerve burnout; exhaustion; stomach irritants and toxins; indigestible toxic foods; diet; anxieties; worries and decreased blood flow.

Heart: Nutrient starvation; circulation impediments; liver congestion; blood alkalosis; glycemia; gluten excesses; hardening of the arteries; allergy vascular spasms and deficiencies; low vitamins E, C, potassium, calcium, magnesium; sudden heart overloads because of stress, grief, loss, anger, frustrations, exhaustion, lack of exercise and an excessive sedentary lifestyle.

Cancer: The problems are far more complex and numerous. Damages to the tissues and cells are very serious and enzymes deficiencies are severe.

Year after year, those with cancer have piled cause upon cause. Over the years their bodies overload with toxins and each one adds to and interacts with the others. Finally, the day comes when the body can no longer take it. The excesses and overloads, the negligence and deprivations, the stresses and abnormalities break down the body's resistance and allow the carcinogens to mutilate and destroy the normalness of cells and transform them into rapid-growing, life threatening cancer cells and tumors.

Tumors are warnings that a body is oversaturated with virulent toxins and poisons. They warn us of the seriousness of our situation and they tell us that we are violating the laws of nature.

Cancer can be a slow gradual health decline, like a gentle slope downwards. The negative forces and attackers have only a small advantage over the cell defenders and body resistance. In this case, a minor preponderance of cell-denaturing forces create only a slow health decline and slow tumor growth. Changes in diet, lifestyle or attitudes and a few, simple remedies; for example, a few mild doses of radioactivity or chemotherapy may be all that is needed to counteract minor causes and stop, and reverse the progress of a cancer tumor growth.

In such cases, simple remedies, as long as they accurately correspond to a patient's needs and problems, can bring about a cure. Unfortunately, such measures have been touted as 'cures' of cancer. They were cures only for those individuals on a slight decline.

What happens when health is on a steep decline?

No one simple, single remedy can or will effectively slow down the cancer processes or rapid growth of tumors. In such cases, simple remedies or approaches such as diet and supplements are not powerful or specific enough to counteract the force or numbers of invaders. Only intense, multiple, long-term, individually-tailored, complete cause-destroying remedies or systems can halt the onslaught of multiple carcinogens.

What about Tumors?

Let's take a look at what tumors are to gain a perspective on why cancer can become a battle for many cancer patients. Tumors are cells that proliferate rapidly and wildly. When multitudes of them have been procreated, the mass they form together becomes palpable and recognized as a tumor.

The processes that create cell growth and proliferation are no different from what happens in our bodies when they create deposits of fatty tissues.

I. People who overeat for many years, indulging in up to twice as much food per day as their bodies need.

II. Much or most of the food they eat is high calorie, fat, fried, refined, overcooked, dead and junk foods, foods that are chemically processed and treated with chemical food additives.

III. Dietary excesses are inadequately eliminated.

IV. Over the years, fatty tissues develop and eventually an accumulation of billions of fat cells grow in size. In a sense, they resemble tumors.

V. Fatty deposits (tumors) do not destroy, kill or harm the body or its organs.

VI. Drugs or specific therapies may slow down or stop the buildup of fatty tissues, but do not successfully rid the body of them.

VII. Starving the body of excesses, which created the fat in the first place, is about the only effective way to melt away the fat.

VIII. A return to dietary excesses regenerates the same fatty tissues. The fat (tumors) comes back.

As long as there is an abundance of enzymes in the stomach, pancreas and intestines that function efficiently, and as long as the liver and intestines process and eliminate the abnormal wastes and excesses, there is no absorption or depositing of these into fatty tissues or putting on weight.

However, no one can overload and overwork their body for years and years and expect it to keep functioning as it should. There comes a time when the excess food indulgences deplete the liver and the digestive organs. Secretions of the digestive enzymes decrease and foods can no longer digest perfectly.

Gradually, abnormal forms of foods force their way through the intestinal walls and permeate the blood, body fluids and tissues. If the fluids in which the cells bathe are saturated with wastes and excesses, the cells will eventually absorb some of the food and waste excesses. The molecules of these substances will replace normal cell molecules, which eventually will become storehouses of fat.

It is not unreasonable to believe that a body that handles excess waste in a wise and effective way would handle carcinogens any differently. If we accept this, we should also accept that:

I. The toxins poison the muscles of the intestinal walls and impair their ability to contract and force out the fecal matter.

II. Tumors are created by poisons that have not been properly processed and handled by our body's metabolism.

III. Cancer cells' membranes are unable to block the absorption of environmental substances. The greater amount of poisons that surround them, the faster and the more they swell.

IV. The poisons that infiltrate damaged cells destroy the chromosomes and oncogenes that control normal cell growth and multiplication. This allows the cells to grow wildly and out of control.

V. Tumors are normal cells, which have been denatured by the poisons they have absorbed. The tumor cells have become a storehouse of body poisons and carcinogens.

VI. The greater the amount of poisons, the greater the number of cells, which become transformed into poisonous cancer cells, the greater and even the faster is the tumor growth.

VII. Tumors could be compared to gangrene. Something either seriously damaged and poisoned a tissue or cut off the circulation to it, and from this tissue, created conditions like a swamp. If not corrected, and blood is not allowed to freely flow, the swamp of toxins will eventually seep back into the system of poison in the rest of the body. This can kill. In cancer, the swamp becomes a tumor.

We can reasonably deduce that tumors are not the body's mistake. Nature does not make mistakes. Mistakes are made by those who knowingly or unknowingly allow abnormal chemicals and body-destroying forces to invade their systems. Tumors are the body's wisdom at work and they are the last attempt to protect us from the effects of poisons and carcinogens. They are indications that your body still has an ability to fight the poisons and fight for your life. However, it also says that your fight for life is in its last phase. This is your last chance to get rid of the poisons, or the poisons will get rid of you. Tumors are red flags, warning the body of danger. Tumors are a call for us to:

- Eliminate hazards to our health and life.

- Change our lifestyle, attitudes and mindsets.

- Become a student and a lover of life.

Tumors are beneficial, life-protecting agents. Tumors are friends and boons, not life-threatening monsters that must be destroyed at all costs.

Our body's reactions are encoded into our genes. Some call it innate wisdom. Genetic scientists are saying the same thing when they claim that staggering amounts of information are encoded in the DNA of our cells. This coding creates instant, perfect, life-protecting reactions. Examples of such reactions are:

- A hand over a flame. Messages from our brain rapidly jerks the hand to safety.
- When we sit on a tack the whole body reflexes into a rebound and jumps up and away.
- A poisoned meal triggers the intestines to rapidly rid the body of the contamination by means of diarrhea.
- Our body will periodically throw off excessive toxic wastes by way of a mucus flushing we call a cold.
- Developing a fever will burn up other toxic excesses.
- The thymus glands and their special white blood cells immediately attack viruses.
- Strong chemical stimuli sends a warning to our brain by creating sensations of pain.
- Strenuous and stressful conditions activate the heart to beat faster and provide more blood, nutrients and life force to handle those situations.

- A pebble in the nose prompts the tissues to secrete a fluid to protect them.
- An object flying in the direction of the head creates reflexes, which makes the whole body jerk away. If coming towards an eye, the eye will instantly close.

Evidence that the body creates tumors as a normal and beneficial, protective procedure is born out of observing tumors initially increasing in size as a result of remedies that later succeed in curing.

Rene Caisse, while treating thousands of cases of cancer, frequently observed over a period of close to 20 years that tumors initially grew larger instead of shrinking as one would normally expect, before receding and eventually disappearing from the benefits of her herbs.

What is also known is that many people, by eliminating and controlling the causes of their tumors, experience a return to health while the tumors stabilize, neither growing or receding. A solid fibrous wall is built around the tumor, which blocks its re-absorption. However, this can be a dilemma. With our conditioned beliefs that tumors are evil, most cancer victors will cling to anxieties, continuing to live in fear by believing the tumor is a possible murderer. This is a serious impediment to healing.

If a body no longer needs the tumor, why does it not reabsorb and disappear? If it does not, what is the right approach to handling it? Is it not best to always destroy it to get rid of it? We will answer these questions in the next chapter.

CHAPTER 3:
TUMOR MANAGEMENT

Tumors play an important role in cancer, but are not the real evil as we are led to believe. Dr. Leo Roy, MD, ND

1. Destroying Tumors

Lethal drugs and chemotherapy are adding more poisons to a body that is already seriously overloaded. There is no longer the ability to antidote and neutralize those poisons. Surgical removal also involves anesthetics and painkillers, and in both approaches, add insult to injury - neither healing the body nor the cancer's original causes. Tumors play an important role in cancer, but are not the real evil as we are led to believe. It does not seem logical to promptly resort to methods that, while they get rid of the tumor, also do considerable and often serious harm to the body as a whole.

It is not possible to disintegrate tumor cells without those cells pouring back the killer poisons into our systems where they have been storing. These poisons will again saturate tissues and again threaten the life of the body. This can start the whole cancer process and cycle all over again. It doesn't seem reasonable to do this without first preparing the body for treatments by increasing the body's ability to handle, detoxify and eliminate them.

Now, there are times when ridding our body of tumors is healthy and lifesaving. Large tumors contain large amounts of toxic, lethal poisons and we need to get rid them. To leave large tumors in our body is like leaving an abscess inside. Abscesses constantly filter their poisons back into, and throughout the whole body and block health restoration. They could possibly revive the whole cancer process.

The best approach to this dilemma would be to totally detoxify the body so that all tumor-creating agents are eliminated. It may take six-12 months to free it of all its toxins. Then, take the tumor out surgically. Doctors who have followed this approach note that almost invariably there is no reoccurrence of tumors. Tumors usually reoccurred in almost all cases when patients underwent surgery too early in panic or fear, discarding the causes and not detoxifying.

More important to keep in mind is patients have no assurance that they will remain tumor free, if they return to their old ways of living, continue to neglect their health and take in body pollutants.

2. Metastases

Let's first define what metastases are. They are secondary malignant growths that develop a distance away from the mother tumors and force their way into blood vessels or lymphatic canals, and travel to other parts of the body. What applies to tumors also applies to metastases, since poisons that created the tumors are already in every area of our body. What is there to stop them from forming tumors anywhere the tissues are susceptible? Tumors can start in any part of the body at any time. The appearance of tumors in other areas than the site in which they first appeared, does not inevitably mean that they are metastases in the accepted meaning of the word. They can be eruptions of cell growths in areas where the cell resistance is the lowest, oxygen and nutrition the poorest, and circulation the most sluggish, and where carcinogens create a pool of body toxin, same as in the primary tumor.

Alternative methods of dealing with tumors

The proper way of handling tumors will be discussed in more detail later. However, it cannot be repeated too often.

Curing Cancer is:

- Detoxifying
- Caring
- Eliminating causes
- Controlling the cancer processes
- Correcting weaknesses and deficiencies
- Restoring total body nutrients
- Saturating bodies with all agents of healing
- Relieving distresses

Most important in healing is not to treat tumors, but to detoxify and restore healing abilities to the whole body.

CHAPTER 4:
DIAGNOSIS: CANCER

At any given moment you have the power to say this is NOT how the story is going to end. Unknown

When we hear the word cancer, it almost inevitably triggers the specter of fear and death. People tend to fall prey to that which they are scared of and the very illness they fear, overcomes them. The prospect of dying creates panic. Much of the panic experienced by patients stem from stories or personal encounters with cancer in others. More importantly, a great deal of what patients feel are the vibrations they pickup from the inner feelings and attitudes of the doctors who are treating them.

Fear is a reaction to the unknown and the fear of cancer, like all fears, results from ignorance. Fear is a measure of a lack of faith: faith in our body's innate wisdom, faith in its healing ability, faith in ourselves and our determination to live; even faith in the power from above that gives us innate wisdom and healing abilities.

In many respects, cancer is an emotional and joy-deficient disease. We need time to play, to enjoy, to appreciate the happiness of life. Joy, play and laughter in life are more than just pleasant moments and activities. They create attitudes that generate a great deal of energy for healing.

When our lives are filled with repression, frustration and suppressions, and we hold on to demoralizing, self-destructive states of mind and powerful self-killing emotions, such as anger, hatred and self-hatred, they yield destructive emotions that damage our overall health and wellbeing. The same goes for mismanaged stress, created by inner conflicts. Continuous emotional conflict leads to fear, anger and guilt, which leads to feelings of helplessness, hopelessness and depression – a short step to despair. Ongoing mental anguish suppresses the organs' functions by which our body eliminates poisons and cancer. Toxic states of mind are another form and way of dying.

Unfortunately, most cancer patients do not nourish their inner being. Without positive attitudes and beliefs, determination and hope and authentic feelings to use as weapons against cancer, the inner environment of the person can be just as toxic as exposure to a lethal physical agent.

Emotions are feelings we choose and determine to experience for ourselves. For example:

- *Negative emotions depress my immune system. Positive ones enhance it.*
- *Negative thoughts and decisions depress my resistance to disease. Positive thoughts and decisions increase immunity and resistance.*
- *I can stop my mind and emotions and listen to what they say. I can learn to:*
  - *Recognize my reactions to the tragedies and difficulties in my life.*
  - *Identify how they influence the onset of my cancer.*
- *A great conqueror of any disease, including cancer is love – non-judgmental, unconditional love.*

Our feelings, attitudes and emotional experiences bear the same relation to the mind that food does to the body. Both mind and body provide sustenance. Each must undergo a process of digestion to be used. What is not useful and used in both must be ultimately discharged. What is held inside, repressed, not faced-up-to realistically, can and does become toxic to the mind and body.

Feelings lead us to hope, cooperation and life, or to despair, rejection and death. Negative feelings can kill. If the ways in which we fall ill, and possibly kill ourselves is to be transformed from chaos into clear understanding, feelings must be considered. When feelings are used as a weapon against someone or ourselves, it can be as toxic as exposure to a lethal physical agent.

We live in a world of relationships and they are an emotional environment. Cancer patients have usually lived in relationships that have had a serious, negative impact on their lives.

The mind influences our biological and emotional states. Even our blood chemistry changes through our contact with others and through the feelings that we are exposed to. Cancer patients are characterized as blockers to themselves.

In most cases, a person diagnosed with cancer erects a false self to hide their malignant thoughts and feelings. They attempt to function as though these thoughts and feelings do not exist and appear normal. The adult personality who is prone to cancer is inordinately pleasant and not prone to aggression or anger. They are anxious to please others.

The most powerful destroyer of a person's defense infrastructure is a traumatic loss. The psychological poisons accumulate and penetrate the cells and activate a chemically-specific vibration that de-nurtures the chromosomes, which controls access to cell growth.

To prevent a psychosomatic cancer from developing, the defensive structure that a person has so carefully constructed needs to be broken down and physiological or psychological carcinogens eliminated.

What to expect from effective healing

Healing is not a reality until all damaged, toxic cells have been replaced by healthy ones. If the replacement process was to start working in the early stages of a therapy, this could take a minimum of two years. However, since the damaging and nurturing of cells will go on as long as the causes and poisons are not completely controlled and eliminated, the cell replacement process may take six, 12 or 20 months – whatever time it takes to complete the body's detoxification. This says that healing is not complete and the cancer process that threatens the patient may not be eliminated for up to three years.

Reasonable Expectations: Treating Symptoms Only

We have been so conditioned by the medical profession to expect relief and improvement of symptoms, as soon as we start on our prescribed therapy. This is only true about the treatment of symptoms. It should be obvious that if the conditions that caused the disease are allowed to continue to exert their will (effects on the body that merely relieve their symptoms without touching the disease causes), the body is not going to be cured.

You can compare symptoms therapy to treating the smoke of a fire. The smoke is merely a symptom of the fire and usually the remedy for such a system is a fan. Nothing works more effectively or quicker. However, in getting rid of the smoke, it also fans the fire to greater fury. In similar ways, treating tumors can bring relief, but fan the cancer process into greater severity. Treating causes often takes time, so one should not expect tumors or the other distresses of cancer to disappear until they have been eliminated.

Premature Hope and Anticipation

Periods of great improvement and feeling wonderful can be deceiving. There is a sense of false security that leads you to believe that your condition has reached a stage where treatments are no longer required and there will be little harm to lessen caring for your body, mind and emotional needs.

It is imperative to remember that you cannot cut back on nourishing your body, mind and emotional needs. You cannot cheat on yourself, your diet, or on your life. You cannot go back to a lifestyle of excess, negative attitudes and emotions, poor habits, nor to the same home or environment of pollutants and expect that your illness will not return or get worse. The return to the abnormalities of your former living will exact the same price tag. Your body is far more sensitive after a period of illness than during the years prior to the illness. In spite of taking the most miraculous cancer cures, and the best possible healing programs, returning to your old ways will not always work.

Chances of a Complete Cure

Only a therapy that accurately and completely provides your total needs, normalizes an abnormal lifestyle and habits can get rid of all carcinogens and causes. If only following parts of your healing needs, you probably won't make it.

Healing is how you live your life. The magic key to curing cancer and cancer prevention is to live - to really live - to live intensely, to live a life full of vigor and hope - to live the true, vital force within you – to discover the real you – to live your truth, completely and totally you.

Reoccurring Tumors

When cancer tumors re-occur the second or third time, they are more difficult to bring under control. Cure failures are now doubled and tripled. The problem is no different than curing a person of poisoning. We know how important it is to flush the poisons out immediately for success and save a life. But when poisons are left in the body, they destroy tissues and erode the body's defenses, and depletes its reserves of healing powers. Poisons left over a period of a year or years, doesn't give the body's defense mechanisms much hope of surviving the poison. On top of that, leaving poisons that are considered genetic, inevitably will continue to undermine vitality and health in the same way.

Ridding the body of tumors while leaving causes to form, is like playing Russian Roulette: the possibilities of curing the cancer and stopping the recurrence of tumors constantly declines over the years.

The amount of therapy required for effective results are greatly increased and the time it takes to obtain the results are significantly prolonged.

Your doctor got it all, but the cancer came back

When we are told that the cancer tumors came back, they really did not. Tumors re-occur, because the real disease was never cured in the first place. The causes of the original tumor and the body processes that created them were not brought to light, treated or managed. If nothing is done to get rid of the tumor causes, inevitably they are still present in the body. Regardless of what therapy was used to destroy the tumors, it won't work as well, as time goes on.

It may take months or years for the dormant cancer cells to multiply and develop into sizes big enough to be felt as tumors. When the *causes* are still there, expect the tumors to rear into existence again.

Spontaneous Remissions

There is no such thing as a "spontaneous remission". Nothing happens without a cause. Spontaneous remissions result from concerted, determined, efforts that succeeded in getting rid of enough of the causes to sufficiently overcome the cancer. Remission results from the effective activities on the part of the organs that detoxify and heal. They have succeeded in overpowering the cancer-causing poisons.

It has often been known that those who change their lifestyle, diet and attitudes, avoid excesses that overload their lives, avoid toxic foods, cigarettes, alcohol, toxic environments, lighten their workloads, responsibilities and or activities, change their attitudes, eliminate excesses, and decide to really live what years they have left, have experienced remissions of their tumors.

Those who determinedly decide that they are not going to die and take whatever measures needed to live right, often succeed. None of it was spontaneous. It was just done without surgery, chemo or radiation. Such successes in overcoming cancer, proves that our minds are more powerful than our bodies, chemistry, drugs, chemo, radiation and surgery. Bodies can work more effectively than they do. Our bodies have means, agents, processes and powers to cure cancer.

Periods of Lows, Reactions and Difficulties

Distressful low periods do not always mean that you are not healing – that you are getting worse. They usually mean that you are healing too fast. You are dumping excesses of disease-causing poisons too quickly back into your blood and into your organs of detoxification. These poisons come in contact with and irritate the nerves, including the nerves of your brain. Of course, you will feel worse. This may well be the 'worst' that is coming out rather than declining body health and that healing is active.

Because there are reverses of feelings of well-being, such times are often called 'healing crises'. They are not really crises. Low periods of apparent failures of healing also mean:

- You have not detected or eliminated at least one of the causes of your illness. It is still affecting and upsetting you.
- There are still external stresses, anxieties, fears or other negatives that are overloading your body beyond its abilities to handle them.
- You may have prematurely cut back on needed treatment and care.
- Maybe you were lax and careless and allowed yourself to go back to old habits or excesses. Or you cheated.
- You may be overloading your body with too many therapies. They are stressing and overworking your body's healing abilities. Treatments need to be cut back over the months. As they saturate the tissues, the intake of large amounts required at the start of treatments are no longer needed in those same amounts. Your improved wellbeing says the same. Your healing program needs to be decreased and kept in harmony with your lesser body needs. Give your body a chance to rest and to catch up with all the energies used to fight the disease and healing.

Presumptions During Healing

- Many people have overcome cancer. Generally, each cancer patient expects to be one of these.
- Treatments can be selected by guesswork.
- Treating tumors is treating cancer.
- When the tumor is gone, the cure is complete.
- Treatments work regardless of the body's states and specific needs.
- Cancer can be cured by the mere taking of anti-cancer remedies and supplements.
- Detoxifying the body and ridding it of carcinogens is of minor importance when taking supplements and remedies that indicate what my body needs.
- Treatments work regardless of body toxicity.

- Vitamins, minerals, amino acids are capable of curing cancer without their team of enzymes.
- A treatment that has cured someone else's cancer will cure mine.
- Herbs are excellent cures for cancer.
- All herbs always work, regardless of the body's state or toxicity.
- Herbal remedies, from whatever sources, are of equal value.
- Once the tumor and all symptoms of cancer are gone, one can safely cut back and cut out the cancer therapy.
- Chemicals and chemical-type therapies can cure cancer.
- Having the belief that as long as a reliable cancer treatment is faithfully followed, health will automatically be restored and the tumors will go away, and not come back. It can happen, but only when your body's healing powers, resistance and immunity have been restored to a point where it is able to rid of the main causes of cancer – the carcinogens and poisons.

Healing cancer requires change, work, patience, and perseverance. Fighting off toxins and poisons is stressful to the body and causes a lot of work for the organs that detoxify and eliminate. They can eventually tire out. What was assumed to be a complete cure and success, often rebuilds the general health of only the body, without attacking the cancer itself.

Healing is not a casual pastime nor a spectator sport. It is a function of personal responsibility and involvement.

As you begin to experience feeling better consistently, do not build up high hopes of being over your troubles. Problems are not over until healing is complete. Prematurely putting aside remedies and healing needs can result in improvements slowing and gradually being replaced by declining health.

Presumptions about Cancer Remedies

Curing by systems

Patients do not fit into generalized, pre-prescribed curing "systems". The therapies for healing must be customized and tailored to suit the needs of each patient. Even their program of treatment(s) must consistently be monitored to ensure they are in harmony with the patient. Those therapies may need to change from month-to-month, as they correct problems and carcinogen levels decline, and cells and tissues are restored. One definition of health that must not be neglected is: balance.

Chemotherapy

Chemotherapy destroys local tumors. It inhibits or delays the growth of deficient cells, but only for a short period of time. It also seriously poisons the whole body, decreasing its resistance to the disease. Its side effects are so drastic that the amounts that can be used in hopes of destroying tumors is very limited. Chemotherapy is not new. It is a replay of our efforts to kill tumors in past centuries by the uses of other poisons like arsenic and heavy metals.

Herbal Remedies as Cures

There are a number of misleading assumptions about the effectiveness of herbs as a "cure". Many herbal customers read on the label a list of herbs known to cure cancer and believe there is a guarantee that they will. Scientists, whose job is to evaluate the healing qualities of herbal remedies, state that the content of healing elements and their effectiveness can vary from five to 95 percent.

Active and healing ingredients in herbs are the multitudes of enzymes their cells create. Enzymes that perform specific physiological functions do so only because they have absorbed special trace minerals from the soil, which make specific healing abilities possible. For example, you may have heard of the Essiac Herbs to cure cancer. The original Essiac herbs were from the Hudson Bay Shield Mountain Range of the middle to northern

Ontario, Canada. The soils were abundantly rich in specific minerals those herbs needed, and such, they healed.

The same herbs harvested in mineral depleted soils, used to make the same Essiac Formula (Florida or many areas of the plains), do not successfully cure cancer. Herbs that are old and stale lose their life force, and their enzymes degenerate and decay the same as do foods. They become useless as herbal healers.

Many assume that taking herbs in any form or preparation automatically heal. Yet, any good herbalist knows that many of the healing agents of herbs can be made available and capable of healing only if extracted first by alcohol.

"Essiac" Herbs

There is an assumption that the Essiac herbs is a four-herb formula and it is promoted as such. This is the formula patented and registered with the Canadian Health Protection Agency – an equivalent to the US FDA. The Essiac Formula was patented because of the persecution by medical drug companies. Rene Caisse – creator of the formula – realized that making the whole formula known would be its death knell; the herbs would be blacklisted and made unavailable to anyone. She guarded this formula with her life.

She gave the formula to no one, including doctors and friends, and those she worked with. There was no one who could guarantee its protection, its assured availability and distribution to all who needed it. Before dying, she did sell it to one organization: The Respirin Foundation. This organization, now called Essiac International, continues to market it. It is the only company that has the original formula.

Those who use Essiac do so with presumptions. They assume that the herbs, which effectively cured so many diseases 50 years ago, still perform the same 'miracles'. It is in the nature of herbs to normalize natural, physiological and biochemical conditions. However, herbs are not able to counteract the deadly effects of powerful drugs, chemicals or radiation. On the contrary, they destroy the active healing agents of herbs.

Rene Caisse observed that her Essiac Formula worked very poorly or not at all when used by people taking any other forms of chemical treatments, be it vitamins or minerals, or drugs. It rarely succeeded in curing those who had undergone radiation or chemotherapy therapy. Surely every good herbalist will confirm this observation.

There is a way to overcome the differences of the times and the pollutants of civilization. Putting patients through a program of intense detoxification, fasting, enemas, detoxifying supplements, liver flushes, sometimes chelation therapy, hydrotherapy, homeopathic detoxification, etc., can succeed in restoring many or most people to a state somewhat similar to the health of people 50 years ago. After months of such a program, many patients will benefit from the Essiac herbs. Their curing powers again become effective.

A common mistake and assumption is believing that our body will respond to a specific cure, because many other peoples' did; for example, believing that remedies like vitamins, minerals, enzymes, proteins, special diets, fasting and various systems like Laetrile or Essiac are universal remedies that guarantee cures. The chemistry and healing abilities of our body are as different as are our appearance and body shape. Before there will be a cancer cure for any individual, there will have to be as many formulae as there are human beings.

For patients to not know what is happening, why it is happening to them, how to control, eliminate and manage what is happening, is a severe stress. Then, to be treated with obscure and especially negative, no-hope-type terminology, the stress is often strong enough to block all their body's abilities to heal. Most patients, just knowing this, have a much easier time of accepting such answers than no answers at all, or answers that lead only to dead-end streets and death. Patience and moral support are prime requisites in activating their healing abilities.

Patients should never become pessimistic

A doctor's honesty should restore their patients' morale and rid them of fatalism and giving up hope. Cancer should not be explained and treated as if it were any other disease. Patients must learn to realize that more than one treatment will probably have to be administered and that it will take a much longer time, and more treatments than those that successfully overcome simple diseases.

The next obvious question is: if there are simple, easy, inexpensive and effective treatments that do absolutely no harm to patients, why are our great scientific doctors still limiting their cancer approaches to the standard drugs, cut and burn treatments? I would answer by saying that the principles of their beliefs and practices have been carved into their minds like being carved into stones. They believe:

- Disease is evil.
- Tumors are evil.
- Evil has to be destroyed.
- The only treatments that rid bodies of tumors are drugs, surgery and radiation.
- There is no need to treat the causes of the disease.
- Science does not know the cause of cancer, even though multiple causes are published in scientific books.
- The essence of the cancer treatment is treatment of symptoms – what a patient experiences. But why are patients who overcame the causes of cancer ignored?
- Only medical doctors have the mental ability and the scientific training to enable someone to understand cancer.

Medics in general pay little heed to what is the essence of both cancer research and cancer therapies.

Research and therapy are totally controlled by the cancer societies, the National Institute of Health and the FDA; the chemical and drug companies and the hospital associations, and by financial interests, which raise over a billion dollars a year in the US alone.

Health Restorers

Since cancer always results from the action of multiple causes combined, working together to achieve a cure requires the control and elimination of all hazards, poisons and all other causes, plus the complete restoration of all nutrients and life force – everything that is required for optimal health. The execution of these curative measures is brought about by the following:

Liver Restoration. There is no healing except by the liver. It is not possible to have cancer with a healthy liver.

Liver Detoxification. The liver is the main organ for handling, neutralizing, detoxifying, breaking down and flushing out poisons and body waste. Without a normal liver, a body cannot rid itself of the causes of cancer, nor of its tumors.

Bile. The liver cannot dump its poisons into the intestine for elimination except by being dissolved in and carried out of the body by bile.

Pancreas. A healthy pancreas perfectly digests foods and sustains our body's immunity on a high level. It is a powerful tumor dissolver that digests and disintegrates all the abnormal, dying, toxic, damaged and devitalized cells, including cancer cells.

Stomach enzymes and hydrochloric acid. Most serious diseases start in the stomach when it fails to secrete needed amounts of stomach enzymes and hydrochloric acid. 95 percent of cancer patients lack these digestive juices.

Thymus. Thymus hormones exert specific anti-cancer actions. Much of them help to increase the drainage of body toxins through the lymphatic channels. Lymph nodes procreate white blood cells that scavenge body toxins and waste. They destroy toxic bacteria and viruses.

Thyroid. The thyroid hormones mostly accelerate all the biochemical activity of our bodies. This is a major factor in burning up and getting rid of poisons and protecting the body against their damaging effects.

Body Immunity and Resistance. Every organ, tissue, cell, force and biochemical function contribute to protecting our body from invaders and from harm – including cancer.

Vitality and Life Force Resources. As cancer is a form of cells dying, every revitalizer helps prevent it. We maintain these forces by a lifestyle of moderation, foods which are alive and fresh in enzymes, by magnetic forces, relaxation, rest, exercise, the joys of living and sleep. Healing only takes place while sleeping.

Correct all deficiencies of enzymes, proteins, oils, vitamins, minerals and trace minerals.

Detoxification Practices
Possibly the most effective way to detoxify is by fasting. The best poison-cleansing agents are:

- Bentonite, psyllium seed, flaxseed and bran.
- Enemas, be they water, coffee, or oil retention.
- Herbal detoxifiers: some of the better ones are burdock, dandelion, milk thistle, and concentrated beets in tablet form.

Letting go. Releasing anxieties, fears, angers, negative emotions, memories and hurts of the past.

Avoiding excesses. Overloads, responsibilities, work, play, TV, including excesses of inactivity.

Positive attitudes. Learning and/or adopting self-love (not self-centered love), self-appreciation, self-esteem and self-confidence.

Eliminate and reject: Negative influences, attitudes, friends, associates, lifestyles, ways of living.

Resolve grief, stresses, tensions: Use the services of a good counselor or friend, if necessary.

Make generous use of known protectors against cancer:

- Flax, sunflower and sesame seed oils
- Laetrile-rich foods: almonds, apricot seeds, seed foods
- Shark and beef cartilages
- Cruciferous foods: broccoli and green leafy vegetables
- Sprouted wheatgrass - juiced or freeze dried tablets
- Fresh, alive, raw or undercooked foods
- For most people a predominantly vegetarian type diet

The best treatment for cancer is cancer prevention.

Predictions about a survival time like, *"you only have three months to live"*, is misleading and cruel, and used to instill fear. No such prediction or prognosis should ever be given to anybody on this basis alone.

Any experienced doctor, having evaluated the lack of health of a patient and the severity of the condition, could make a reasonable estimation about how long a patient can live, if he or she were given known doses of drugs that poison or treatments that shorten life.

However, if we were to disregard such morbid negativism – uncover every possible cause of the disease, every weakness of the body, everything that is lacking that could shorten our survival time, then correct and eliminate those causes, stop poisoning and damaging the body and its organs; stop anything that will shorten our days and provide the body, mind, spirit, and soul with all their needs, nutrients, energy sources, vitality reserves and morale builders, leave nothing to chance, cover and control every problem, who is there on this earth that can predict the years left for any cancer patient to live?

As a rule of thumb, it is not unreasonable to expect at least double the time left to live, predicted by death-instrument-using doctors. However, given that time, the body has a chance to recuperate its healing and living abilities. What starts as only double survival time can possibly be quadrupled. If the quadrupled time is within the range of two years, it is possible that a body can disintegrate and eliminate all the sick cells, and replace them with new healthy ones. It is not impossible. Generous years of ongoing living are also possible.

The death sentence of incurable merely means that:

- Few or none of the causes of your cancer are pinpointed and clarified.
- All causes of the disease are not treated. If not known, of course, they will not or cannot be treated, managed, or eliminated.
- Only drugs, surgery, synthetic chemical remedies, chemotherapy are included as therapies.
- Nothing is included in the healing program that will restore or rebuild the body's resistance to disease.
- Only remedies which damage the body: surgery, chemo and radiation destroy the body's healing abilities.
- Remedies which are known to cause cancer are used at the same time as remedies that are healers.

Under these conditions, no cure is possible. No one has to settle for such conditions.

The cure of any and every disease is living, restoring life, restoring the life forces and all the nutrients and elements that promote life and make life possible.

You cannot, or do not die until you make a decision that you want to die or accept death.

This is emphatically spelled out in the following story of attitude told by Norman Cousins, American author of *Anatomy of an Illness*:

The doctor entered the room of an 81-year-old lady and commenced to tell her that the reports of her rasps indicated cancer and that she would be best to get her affairs in order for there is nothing anyone could do for her, especially at her age. She walked up to him looked at him in the face, eyeball to eyeball and said F – you. Could the vulgar phrase better express her positive attitude and determination to live?

Eight years later the same doctor, walking down a hall of the same cancer department, noticed her talking to and assisting cancer patients on the ward.

Intimately knowing the personality, idiosyncrasies and often strange ways of healing processes will add greatly to your hopes, confidence and healing abilities.

Pain Control

All pain is caused by irritants that contact nerve endings. The job of nerves is to transmit messages to the brain, telling it that abnormal conditions are present in an area of the body. The irritant can be a pressure, excess heat, cold, acids or alkaline. Ninety five percent of the irritants, which cause pain to our bodies are poisons. The greater amount of poisons and the greater the toxicity of those poisons, the more severe the pain.

Caffeine either by direct injection into the bloodstream or by intake, via the rectum, can control pain. This is one reason why it is contained in most headache pills.

When absorbed in the colon, the caffeine flows directly to the liver. It stimulates the liver in the same way as it does our nerves. The chemical stimulation activates the liver to flush out large amounts of its residual toxins and then eventually those from the body.

The answer to pain control is poison control. Total detoxification can relieve pain that even morphine will not.

A doctor can alter a patient's pain threshold by the use of serotonin, a natural chemical that acts on the brain. Dr. Simon Seltzer, Temple University School of Dentistry, Philadelphia.

Enzymes are our body's painkillers. By detoxifying, enzymes are the major control agents of pain.

Detoxification may require taking enemas or colonics until the pain is completely relieved. In extreme pain, such as in terminal cancer, many enemas may be needed. Each colonic can flush out as much intestinal poisons as four to six enemas.

Taking enemas may not relieve distresses or pain until the intestines and liver are thoroughly cleansed of their poisons. It may take five to 15 or more to do this. For example, enema number 10 or number 12 may do nothing, but after enema number 13 or more, the body experiences a breakthrough – a sense of relief. It is like the sun coming through a cloud. The pain eases remarkably.

This effect is not permanent. The tissues dump their reserves of poison into the blood and into the liver. The pain will come back, but not so severely. Each successive reoccurrence of pain will require less enemas, but enemas always relieve.

Weight Loss and Emaciation

Weight loss that accompanies cancer does not have to be a severe problem, as so many cancer patients experience it to be. Cancer patients almost invariably lack digestive enzymes, especially those of the pancreas. Their foods do not digest thoroughly as they should. Poorly digested foods cannot be absorbed into or utilized by cells and tissues. Cancer patients can be seriously starving even while eating nutritious and substantial meals. A careful assessment of their digestion will show that this is a big part of their health and cancer problem, and the major reason for their shrinking bodies.

The answer and the solution is of course digestive enzymes. By using the quality and quantities their bodies need, even the most emaciated cancer patient can live to see their body's weight restored, even back to its original normal. Cancer patients can, and possibly always, require more enzymes of their saliva in order to assimilate sugars or more stomach enzymes and hydrochloric acid in order to assimilate the food proteins (95 percent of cancer patients do not secrete sufficient quantities of hydrochloric acid); or more of the pancreatic enzymes in order to digest and assimilate the oils to complete the final stages of transformation of the sugars and proteins into utilizable nutrients.

This does not mean just taking any digestive enzymes, or trying to satisfy digestive needs by guesswork. The specific ones a body requires, and in the right amounts, must be determined and taken properly. There are no fixed amounts of digestive enzymes that satisfy every body's needs. Not taking enough makes about as much sense as phoning a friend and then dialing only dial six out of the seven numbers, then wondering why the phone doesn't work to connect to your friend.

Therapists tend to prescribe amounts of enzymes either according to the label on the bottle or according to their experience. Many patients take them on their own, also using them according to what is on the label and by their own guesswork.

The quantities of digestives needed, will vary according to:

- The ability of the digestion organs.
- The digestibility of the foods and their concentration of nutrient to the quantities of food taken.
- The state of fatigue of the patient.
- The emotional state of the patient, their stresses, tensions, anxieties, worries, will markedly cause contraction of the blood vessels to the organs that create the enzymes and decrease the abilities of the organs to create the amount patients need.

Failure to take all the above conditions into consideration, can account for almost all emaciated cancer patients.

There are simple ways to determine the amounts and kinds of digestive enzymes a patient needs without going through serious, complicated, expensive laboratory and hospital testing.

I. Carefully consider all symptoms of digestion: fullness and bloating after meals, gas by burping or passing wind by the rectum, burning of the stomach, fatigue after meals, abnormal proteins or cramps, loss of appetite or insatiable appetites, cravings for certain foods.

Careful observation of the stool characteristics:

- Less frequent bowel movements after substantial meals.
- Painful bowel movements (hemorrhoids).
- Blood in the stools.
- BM evacuation is possible only by forcing.
- Fibers and undigested foods are visible in the stools.
- Stools are full of holes like sponges, not a smooth surface.
- Stools are fragmented, bits and pieces, not formed like a solid sausage.
- Stools are soft mushy, or hard.
- Stools do not sink, but float on the surface of the toilet water.
- The color is not dark brown, but it is pale brown, yellowish or grayish.
- Foul odor – putrefaction of poorly digested proteins or lack of foul odor, indicating sugar fermentation.

II. Trial and error. Begin using stomach enzymes for a few days. Start with a large amount until there is definite bowel movement improvement. Decrease the amount to a minimum number that still produces maximum relief of symptoms and maximum normalization of bowel movements. Then try the pancreatic enzymes, using them in the same way. After, try both together. It may take a week or two to learn to understand your body's needs. It may take longer to understand the variations of your body's needs, according to diet and lifestyle.

Balancing Herbal Regimes

Herbs, like remedies and healing regimes, also have to be used with discretion and judgment. Throwing various remedies together by guesswork and assumption can often guarantee failure rather than success. Assumptions also misinterpret low periods to mean that the remedies are not right for you, your treatment is not working, or your cancer is not being controlled or overcome.

Nature and Your Healing

Mother Nature and your body are benevolent tyrants. They demand to be consistently treated with justice and consideration. They expect to be appreciated, respected, revered and to be a dominant focus of your life – to be used, but not abused. They handsomely reward those who respect and furnish them with all their needs and cruel to those who are abusive. Yet, they never refuse to heal and repair and restore in miraculous ways – ways beyond our greatest expectations.

Healing is giving nature a real chance.

CHAPTER 5:
CANCER CURING

For so long, the mainstays of cancer treatment have been chemotherapy and radiation. They're toxic and primitive. We need to look at it in a rational way and say, how can we help the body heal itself? Eve Vertes, American Scientist

Curing cancer is...

...detoxifying

...caring

...eliminating causes

...controlling the cancer process

...restoring total body nutrients

...saturating the body with all agents of healing

...relieving distresses

Curing resides with the patient and the function of medicine is merely to activate this process and lend it support. In ignoring the intrinsic gifts for self-repair, a physician obstructs the efficacy of his own scientific methods and impedes the very process of recovery. Bernard Lown, MD, Professor of Cardiology, Harvard University, School of Public Health. From *The Healing Heart* by Norman Cousins.

The Latin word 'cura' means care – not to kill. Health means wholeness. The word 'heal' means to make whole – to restore to its original state of total wellbeing. Healing first involves knowing what needs to be healed. What is the real illness? A first step is to carefully evaluate the state of health of every patient to determine weaknesses, needs, deficiencies, toxicities, the presence of causes of cancer and the effects that these causes have had on the body. Before panicking and throwing reason aside, and starting on a search for a panacea, it is more logical to focus attention on and analyze everything in a patient's environment, lifestyle and nutrition; everything that is not in harmony with his or her nature – everything that is not health-giving and then rid the body of everything that is detrimental, toxic or poisonous.

"Cures" That are Not Cures

As you have noticed, I keep repeating the importance of detoxification. Curing cancer starts with this process. There cannot be a permanent, complete cure without detoxification. To not rid the body of disease causes while applying remedies is futile and doesn't make sense. Poisons react with, neutralize and block the healing processes of even the best remedies. We can better appreciate the importance of this by considering an example: you are eating highly nutritious foods to which a poison has been added. Instead of your body absorbing the nutrients that restores, the poison damages and further poisons.

Nutrients, rest cures, morale rebuilders cannot counteract carcinogens. Nor do simple, single so called 'cancer cures' counteract multiple long-term insidious causes. Resetting, killing, drugging, radiating tumors does not eliminate the invading carcinogens that created the cancer in the first place. These may provide symptom relief. They cannot be considered cures.

Toxins and Body Toxicity

We have been thoroughly conditioned by the chemical companies, polluting industries, drug companies, food companies and medical professions to pay no attention to the multitude of chemicals and pollutants we come in contact with daily. When we succumb to illness, we do not consider the poisons as its cause, or even important. We have been brain-washed into believing that the dosages of poisons and pollutants we live with are so small that they couldn't possibly do us much harm. We believe we are being protected by our Food and Drug Administration (US) or Health Protection Branch (Canada). They would not allow anything hazardous into our food, air, water or environment, *but they do.*

More and more cancer researchers agree that the majority of cancer – perhaps eight or nine out of 10 are caused by substances people chew, inhale, drink or come in contact. There is hardly a moment that we are not in contact or absorbing some of the thousands of toxic chemicals in our environment, food, water and air. The price we pay for assuming that we live in a safe world is illness and even death.

In 1945, the drug companies started dumping chemical fertilizers on to our plants and crops as pesticides and into our foods as preservatives; and into our water and air. In fact, the drugs used by doctors as medication, thousands of tons of poisons and chemicals, were surpluses from the war industry. Unless one lived close to nature and learned to avoid and protect themselves from those poisons, those born since that year (1945) have not spent a single day of their lives without being poisoned. Besides all of the toxins and poisons we absorb from our environment, many more are created and harbored in our bodies. Knowing little about the harmfulness of these poisons and pollutants, few people take precautions to protect themselves or to find ways to eliminate them from their bodies.

We pay no attention to the number of our daily bowel movements. Why should we? Our family doctor constantly assures us that more than one bowel elimination a day is not important; one a day is fine and healthy. This assumption by doctors disregards the whole picture of body pollution. How can it be normal to ingest three good meals a day – to have three quantities of food going into the body and only one quantity of refuse is expelled? Surely the body must eliminate as much as it absorbs. If not, poisons will inevitably accumulate. The amounts retained may reach levels beyond the body's tolerance. An elimination equal to ingestion takes into account only what is needed on a daily basis.

What about the toxins, wastes and poisons that have accumulated in our systems for years and generations? It takes more than the normal number of eliminations to catch up and get rid of the backlog.

Healing cancer becomes possible only when elimination succeeds in decreasing the accumulation of body poisons when there are more daily eliminations than meals. Our experiences as authors are that the majority of cancer patients that fail to overcome their illness are those who pay little attention to detoxification and elimination – who fail to have at least four bowel movements a day – who carefully rebuild their body's health, but fail to get rid of the real cancer, the real healing paralyzers: their poisons.

Body pollution is most deceiving. We cannot visualize the amount of poisons that filter through our bloodstream and saturate our tissues and cells until we are freed from their effects. By reflection, we can compare the difference in vigor, wellbeing and vitality and in the clarity of our mind, emotions and living.

What are Toxins and Poisons?

A poison (according to Webster's dictionary), *"is any agent, which introduced into an organism, may chemically produce any injurious or deadly effect, or exert a baneful influence on, corrupt, pervert, and/or inhibit the activity of a catalyst."*

The key word is catalyst. The Webster definition does not tell us what is the catalyst. Without this understanding, we are still in the dark as to the real nature of a poison or how poisons work. There is only one category of biochemical catalysts in our body: enzymes. A poison is anything that inhibits, uses up or destroys enzymes.

Detoxification

Our body cannot tolerate denatured, devitalized, dead cells or substances, surpluses, or poisons - nothing that is foreign to its individuality and blueprint. This brings into play chemical processes that break down, neutralize and eliminate everything that is not natural to, or harmonious with it.

Curing cancer is more the result of detoxification and elimination from the body than from the remedies that are taken in. Proper detoxification is first and foremost essential to every cancer regime. It can be lifesaving.

In our bodies, there are over 20 organs, systems and chemical processes to detoxify and eliminate poisons. This includes processes that disintegrate and manage cells and tissues, cell debris, waste and toxic poisoned cells. Before cancer poisons can overcome a body, the resistance of body organs and systems must have undergone considerable weakening and jeopardy.

The liver is the most powerful and effective of our systems. It handles, neutralizes, detoxifies, and eliminates most body poisons. As long as our liver is healthy and capable of fulfilling its multitude of tasks, no poison – not even those powerful enough to cause cancer – can gain a foothold and survive long enough or accumulate to levels capable of transforming healthy cells into cancer cells. The liver is assisted by other organs of elimination: the colon, kidneys, lungs, skin and lymphatics.

Our body's gentle art of attacking, disintegrating and getting rid of tumors.

The body normally and consistently destroys any and every cell that is not healthy and strong, every cell that is damaged or dying, every cell that has finished its life's role, every cell that is no longer normal and in harmony with the rest of the body. Twenty seven million cells die each minute – around three billion die each day. Body enzymes normally process all the components of these dead cells and eliminate them from the body. The main enzymes that do this are the same as those that digest the cells of foods that enter the stomach.

There is no vegetable and animal substance that escapes the crumbling action of our stomach and pancreas secretions. They attack and digest the three billion damaged, dying and foreign cells daily, including cancer cells and tumors. Amazingly, they destroy only abnormal cells. They do not touch or affect normal, healthy cells!

The action of digestive enzymes is not solely restricted to digesting foods in the stomach and intestines. These same enzymes travel to every square inch of our bodies. Together with foods, they pass through the walls of the intestines, into the body and blood, and into body fluids.

It is not possible for abnormal, foreign cancer cells to survive contact with these enzymes. Cancer cells succeed in surviving and flourishing only when there are not enough digestive enzymes to attack and destroy them. As long as all organs of digestion – the saliva glands, the stomach, pancreas and liver are strong, healthy and secreting abundantly, it is not possible for cancer cells or those on the way to becoming cancer cells, to escape being destroyed by those enzymes.

Cancer tumors can be treated and destroyed by the use of digestive enzymes instead of using chemotherapy or radiation.

This is not to be construed that digestive enzymes are a cure-all of cancer. They cannot and do not destroy poisons, chemicals and carcinogens. All enzymes, including digestive enzymes, are fragile. They are vulnerable to the destructive actions of drugs and poisons, and are destroyed by them. The poisons that cause cancer also destroy the enzymes that protect cells from being transformed into abnormal cancer cells. They destroy body immunity and resistance to them.

Powerful negative emotions, grief and traumas that predispose and contribute to cancer also burn and deplete our protective enzymes.

Detoxifying and Healing Cautions

It is possible to heal too fast – to break down the tumors, liberate their contents and pour them back into our body too fast – faster than our body's detoxifying and eliminating organs can handle. Going on prolonged fasts or taking large amounts of detoxifying remedies can free too many stored poisons too quickly and overload the liver. Body waste and garbage can overload and plug the liver like a clogged sink's drain. They can saturate and exhaust it and the organs that assist it.

Words of warning: excessive detoxification can leave you feeling as if your treatment is not working, or it is working against you. Exhaustion and depressed feelings can make it worse. Pain may increase. Serious toxic reactions can sometimes last weeks. Most healing crises normally last four to five days.

When such distresses or negative reactions occur, or when any of the above reactions or at the first sense of pain, follow the following recommendations.

Take enemas. Take them often. Take them often enough to completely eliminate the poisons that cause the pain. Keep taking them until the pain is all gone. For at least one day, take five, 10, 15. Do whatever it takes to obtain relief.

Learn to listen to the symptoms, signals and messages your body is experiencing. To avoid or control these unpleasant times:

- Slow down.
- Give your body and detoxifying organs a rest.
- Modify your healing program.
- Give your body time to catch up with the overload.
- Give it time to rid itself of its excess body garbage.
- Periodically and temporarily, even if you feel comfortable and well, give your body a four-to-five-day "Sabbath" from your healing regime.
- Cut way back on all therapies until systems of distress have cleared.
- Decrease or stop taking all those supplements, which according to your prescription chart are indicated for healing and rebuilding the body and its immunity. Healing requires energy and work. There are times when those energies used in healing are needed to handle the surplus of toxins.
- At such times, focus on detoxifying. Increase the number of detoxifying supplements – those which function to activate and support the organs of detoxification and elimination.
- Go back to your healing program later, when the detoxification reaction has subsided.

- If putting aside certain remedies leave you feeling less well, go back to those supplements recommended for the symptoms you experienced. These particular supplements should not be discounted until your healing is well advanced.

Curing multiple causes requires multiple remedies

To win the battle against cancer, there is no single panacea or weapon. In order for therapies to be successful, they must be complete. They must include remedies that:

- Reinforce and protect cells.
- Create and strengthen immunity and resistance.
- Provide in abundance all nutrients, enzymes, vitamins, minerals, etc., that are essential for restoring and re-generating every requirement of cell structures and functions.
- Revitalize, rest, and preserve all energies for healing.
- Neutralize all pollutants and foreign agents.
- Detoxify, purge, cleanse and eliminate.
- Keep everything in the body in harmony and balance.

Therapies must vary and be proportional to the body's needs, according to the severity of disease processes, the status of health progress and changes.

The Carpenters and Builders of Health

Remedies are our biochemical tools and instruments of healing and our body's organs use the tools in the same sense that carpenters and house builders use building materials and work with hammers and saws. The building organs – the carpenters of health for our body – are primarily our liver, stomach and pancreas. The liver is a laboratory of all living. Our stomach and pancreas are organs that render nutrients into a form utilizable by the liver and other organs. The building materials are our nutrients. The tools, which work these nutrients are enzymes. Enzymes are the elements that have the ability to bring about biochemical changes, prepare nutrients, break down toxins and maintain health and healing. Enzymes are the biochemical agents by which our liver and all organs of healing and detoxification function.

It is not possible to succumb to cancer if all the organs, body mechanisms and chemical agents are in good health and function at peak capacity. It makes little sense to expect healing tools and agents to work when the organs, like carpenters who build the house, are in poor health. The best cancer remedies can be rendered ineffective by inadequate functioning of the organs of healing.

Cancer-curing Agents: Our World of Enzymes

Enzymes are our micro-molecular miracle workers – the weavers and sparks of life. There is no other element, substance or chemical in the world or in nature with their abilities or functions.

Enzymes are microscopic, alive catalysts – the agents of all biochemical reactions, of all resisting attackers and invaders. They are our cell protectors and revitalizers. They are responsible for repairing cell breakdowns and abnormalities. Enzymes regulate cell growth and cell multiplying and dividing. They are our body's detoxifying and healing experts. They make possible and maintain every action and function involved in living. They function in every cell, organ and tissue of our body. They created the difference between healthy cells and sick cells – alive cells and dead cells.

There are about a half a million different types of enzymes. Each enzyme is a conglomeration of several thousand – up to 60,000 – of molecules of amino acids. Many thousands of such enzymes are in each of our 70 to 100 trillion cells. Some enzymes, combined with trace minerals, orientate their activities to specific functions.

Enzymes could be compared to microchips in a computer. Computers cease to function when only one chip becomes faulty or taken out of the system. The same with the human body. Enzymes are crucial to life and healing. When cells of our body are depleted of even just one enzyme system, they die. When cancer therapies are devoid of enzymes and cancer patients have depleted all of their reserves of enzymes, even the most miraculous of therapies cannot heal. Other than physical/traumatic injuries, there is no disease that can maintain its existence in our body if our enzyme resources are functioning perfectly.

It is unbelievable that the conspiracy of silence about enzymes, manipulated by the chemical and drug companies has succeeded in almost obliterating our awareness and understanding of enzymes. In so doing, they have created the greatest barrier possible against healing cancer, as well as many other degenerative diseases.

Cancer is a deficiency of many enzymes over many years. The lack of enzymes weakens the abilities to resist and fight disease.

CHAPTER 6:
EMPOWER YOUR OWN HEALING

I really do think that any deep crisis is an opportunity to make your life extraordinary in some way. Martha Beck, Author

I've been seeing many cancer patients in my office and I prefer to begin the consultation with encouraging words:*"Healing their cancer really begins with them – not their doctors or with me and the commitment to do their best to heal is absolutely paramount"*. I also want to ensure that they consult with their doctors throughout my work with them. Healing cancer is a partnership with me, a naturopathic doctor, their medical doctors and with the patient.

First and foremost, healing involves working with the body and with the problem, with carefulness and precision. Sometimes it requires only one negligence, one error, or an essential missing link to block healing. All treatments need to be followed 98 percent of the time. Every degree less than 90 percent, lessens chances of returning to health. Those that follow only 80 percent of what their bodies need may have as little as 50 percent chance of overcoming their cancer.

It is the immunity resistance factors in the body that perform most of the curing. Holistic, effective cancer therapies should restore digestive organs: the saliva glands, liver, stomach and pancreas. The following make up and help body resistance:

- **Restore** organs that detoxify and eliminate: liver, pancreas, spleen, thymus, thyroid, intestines.
- **Restore** body vitality and life forces by the use of live food, sprouts, green life, magnetic therapy, rest, sleep, relaxation.
- **Balance** the endocrine glands: sympathetic, parasympathetic and nervous system.
- **Restore** and maintain balance of body biochemicals: the acids, alkalines and pH.
- **Increase and improve circulation**: eliminate local circulation impediments and blockages through physical exercise and massages after detoxification has been done.
- **Correct deficiencies** by restoring enzymes and with total vitamin complexes and trace minerals, essential proteins, oxygen, and oxygenation.

- **Relieve negative emotions** of stresses, grief, worries, anxieties and fears. Give or accept personal and moral support, and encouragement.
- **Follow a protective diet:** live, undercooked, fresh, natural, organic foods and tea. Supplements, cruciferous foods, good quality protective oils, shark cartilage, beef, herbal remedies: the original Essiac Herb formula.
- **Restore, rehabilitate the organs** that create curing: curing must not be limited to supplying the tools and agents, such as the vitamins, minerals, proteins, and specific biochemical nutrients needed for healing. The organs that use and work these healing agents must also be restored. Like building a house, one doesn't just bring on site building materials. A capable and efficient builder is just as important as the materials and tools.
- **Enlighten yourself** by carefully following guidelines and counsel to avoid all lifestyle and health-depleting excesses.
- **Modify attitudes** through counseling and making life-affirming decisions.

Supplements: Vitamins and Minerals

In addition to a healthy dietary intake, vitamins and minerals are necessary to attain optimum wellness.

Our metabolism is regulated by vitamins that keep our body functioning at high performance levels. They reduce blood pressure and they are critical for immune system support, resistance to infection, protect against heart disease and prevent or help cure many other health problems.

Vitamins are essential nutrients and they are referred to as micro-nutrients, because in comparison to carbohydrates, fats, proteins and water, they are used in comparatively small amounts to maintain and keep the body's biological chemistry functioning properly.

Since vitamins occur naturally in animals and plants, they are called organic compounds. For humans, vitamins act as coenzymes and become integrated into the body parts such as blood, bone, cells, enzymes, hormones and muscles. They are activators or catalysts to create a balanced biochemical state in our bodies. For example, vitamin B6 is needed for the enzyme that triggers nerve impulses to your fingers. A deficiency could result in numbness to your fingers. Without it, the enzyme responsible for making this happen in your body cannot work. These biochemical reactions are constantly occurring in the body, keeping it fine-tuned and ready to deal with the many assaults upon it, such as polluted air and water.

For cancer patients, understanding all the literature expounding the virtues, healing abilities and need for vitamins, minerals, antioxidants, herbs, and a multitude of other remedies can be overwhelming by all. They have been persuaded to believe that curing cancer results more from what they put in their bodies rather than what they get out. The contrary is more realistic, true and successful.

Supplements are very beneficial for those with cancer, but remember, taking supplements into a toxin-riddled body will encounter the poisons that are present, react with them, and be neutralized and destroyed by them. Total body cleansing and avoidance of harmful and unnatural substances are essential. This includes all refined, processed foods and similar type supplements.

The following supplements are beneficial to prevent cancer, but they actually assist with the psychological stress of having the disease and also aid in healing it, once the toxins and poisons have been eliminated from the body through detoxification.

B-Complex vitamins metabolize carbohydrates, fat and proteins, which aid in energy production. They also contain antioxidants, such as vitamins A, C, E and the mineral selenium. They also restore the proper function of our nervous system and reduce damage to our immune system.

In some cases, intramuscular injections are used for quick results, and add to this, liver and B6 (pyrodoxine) injections under the supervision of your doctor. Self-supplementation is possible, using B-complex in pill form with an extra helping of B5 (pantothenic   acid),   the   anti-stress   vitamin.

Magnesium is one of the most beneficial minerals our body needs. Not enough can be said about the importance of this mineral. It is required for enzymatic steps, which food components are metabolized and new substance are produced by the body. In fact, there are about 300 known enzymatic reactions in which magnesium plays a role. For example, magnesium is a cofactor involved in the formation of a compound called *cyclic AMP* (cAMP), which is a necessary step in the cellular response to hormones. This entire system is magnesium dependent, so much so that our body's ability to respond to hormonal signals is affected by magnesium deficiency.

Magnesium is well absorbed from the gut and the colon. This absorption is not affected by the presence of other ions in the diet. Magnesium absorption does not interfere with calcium or phosphate transport from the gut. It regulates the movement of ions in the heart and muscles that are required for maintaining a proper heart rhythm and proper muscle and nerve conductions throughout the body.

Magnesium seems to be able to control the 'set point' cell functions and that is, regulate the various responses of the body to stress. So it is the most critical mineral for managing stress. Magnesium is also required to burn sugar for energy and calms the over stimulation of cells produced by the stress-induced release of calcium.

Vitamin C is water soluble and a powerful antioxidant, which helps scavenge and stabilize free radicals to help lower oxidative stress in the body. It is a factor in the normal development and maintenance of bones, cartilage, teeth and gums. It helps stimulate immune cell functions, wound healing and connective tissue formation.

The minimum daily requirement for vitamin C relates to prevention of scurvy. It is generally agreed that the total body pool size of ascorbate should be at least 900 mg. This is the total amount of vitamin C in the body on any given day. To achieve this level, a daily intake of 30 to 40 mg per day is sufficient. As ascorbate has been shown to be of extremely low toxicity, higher dosages may be consumed. Ascorbic acid is a reducing agent involved with the transfer of electrons from molecule to molecule. In addition to working in a variety of anabolic processes involving the synthesis of new molecules, it has impressive antioxidant activity.

Vitamin C is also needed for *carnitine synthesis*, which is essential for the oxidation of fatty acids. It is also required for the synthesis of neurotransmitters and the detoxification of foreign compounds, via a *mixed function oxidase system*.

Intake of oral vitamin C increases iron absorption and also protects folate and vitamin E oxidative damage in the body.

Clinical Aspects of Vitamin C

A short review of vitamin C's many beneficial actions from an impressive body of scientific literature includes:

- Immune system enhancement. Ascorbate is used by white blood cells during a cold to fight infectious organisms.
- Vitamin C may increase resistance to infection and help the body combat an infection in process.
- Reduction of blood levels of histamine during a cold. Histamine is the molecule that is responsible for many cold symptoms.
- Antioxidant properties. Ascorbate is a scavenger for the superoxide and hydroxyl radicals.
- Like vitamin E, it is associated with protecting the water-soluble components. It also helps reduce deactivation of vitamin E.
- Detoxification of heavy metals and toxic organic compounds such as *benzapyrene* (fromsmoke) or *anthracene* and some pesticides.
- Vitamin C appears to be able to prevent the conversion of sodium nitrate (a meat preservative) into nitrosamines.
- Some clinical trials have shown that vitamin C may reduce clot formation and can protect against early *atherosclerotic*

change in the blood vessel wall. Disorders such as certain hypersensitivity (allergic) reactions are improved by ascorbate administration.

Vitamin D is a fat soluble vitamin. Inadequate amounts of Vitamin D, coupled with insufficient sunlight exposure, can result in Vitamin D deficiency. It helps with overall maintenance of vital organs, regulates calcium and phosphorous levels in the blood and promotes mineralization of bones. Another important fact about this vitamin is that it works synergistically with a number of other vitamins, minerals and hormones. Higher levels of Vitamin D is beneficial since it has been linked to a lower risk of cancers, such as colon, prostrate, breast and lung cancer.

Manufactured from cholesterol in the skin after irradiation with ultraviolet light (sunlight), it can also be ingested orally. This compound is converted by the kidneys into a hormone called 1, 25-dihydroxycholecalciferol. This hormone circulates to the intestine and instructs the cells in the duodenum and jejunum to produce calcium-binding protein. This protein binds with calcium ingested in the diet and transports it into the blood.

Adequate vitamin D in dietary form is required if adequate ultraviolet light is unavailable.

Vitamins E and Zinc are beneficial for proper immune function.

Three other tocopherols present in food are *beta*, *gamma* and *delta* forms of the molecule. There are only minor differences in structure between these molecules, but they have very different activity levels.

Vitamin E functions as an antioxidant. Its main role is to prevent *free-radical induced injury* on the surface of the cell membrane. The cell membrane is made of lipids, which are susceptible to attack by free radicals. Vitamin E quenches these radicals by absorbing them and protecting the cell membrane lipids. For this effect, alpha tocopherol has the highest activity, but all tocopherols have some degree of antioxidant function.

Coronary Artery Disease (CAD) and *intermittent claudication* are both reduced with vitamin E administration. Intermittent claudication is a cramping sensation in the calves which occurs during walking due to obstruction of the arterial supply to the leg.

Enzymes help to break down macro nutrients in foods. They facilitate the millions of biochemical reactions happening every minute. Every cell in the body needs enzymes and each enzyme has a particular job to do. For the body to be able to use carbohydrates, proteins and fats from the foods we ingest, they must be broken down mechanically and chemically in the digestive tract.

Vitamins, minerals, oxygen all need enzymes to make them useful. Without enzymes, plants and animals would not be able to live. It is no different for human beings, as digestive enzymes act as catalysts to breakdown and absorb the nutrients we consume. While they cause change, the enzymes themselves do not change. They convert food into components such as: sugars, amino acids, fats, starches, vitamins, minerals and numerous nutrients like plant phytochemicals. They are the guides that cause the right nutrient to go into the correct cell.

Enzymes of one type cannot be substituted for another type of enzyme. The absence or even a shortage of an enzyme can cause someone to go from a state of health into one of disease or illness.

According to Dr. Anthony Cichoke, author of the book, *The Complete Book of Enzyme Therapy* (Avery Publishing, 1999), enzymes are critical to sustaining life. A lack of enzymes can cause everything from indigestion, allergies, heart disease and a weakened immune system.

Enzymes are categorized according to their purpose in the body. We focus on the digestive enzymes that are known as the hydrolases group and there are four basic digestive enzyme types:

- Amylolytic or amylase, which is in the intestines, pancreas and saliva break down carbohydrates.
- Cellulase breaks down cellulose.
- Lipolytic or lipase breaks down fats.

- Proteolytic or protease in the stomach, intestines and pancreas, break down proteins.

A particular enzyme acts on a specific food component and knows what it is acting on, simply by adding "ase" after the substance. For example, one of the enzymes that acts on sugar is known as sucrose; one that acts on proteins is called protease (also known as "proteolytic enzymes" just to drive us all a little crazy); one that acts on cellulose is called cellulose, and for the milk sugar "lactose" the enzyme is lactase.

Starch-digesting amylase enzymes, alpha-amylase and beta-amylase processes starches into sugars. Alpha-amylase is in the saliva and pancreas. Beta-amylase is in unprocessed raw vegetables and grains. Glucomylase and mylase process starches in the small intestines. They digest thousands of times their own weight in starches. Protein-digesting protease enzymes: bromelain is from pineapple. Pancreatin comes from animal pancreas and works best in the small intestines. Pepsin is from animal enzymes and it breaks down proteins into amino acids. Prolase is from the papain in papaya. Protease is from papaya. Renin takes casein, the milk protein, making it into a usable form for the body and helps release the calcium, potassium, phosphorous, iron and other minerals found in milk. The pancreas also produces chymotrypsin and trypsin to aid in   breaking   down   proteins.

When looking at or purchasing enzymes, here is a sample of the full spectrum of a digestive system enzyme capsule:

- Pancreatic protease, with acid stable protease...breaks down protein.
- Lipase...breaks down fats.
- Alpha amylase...breaks down carbohydrates.
- Amyloglucosidase...breaks down carbohydrates .
- Cellulase...breaks down fiber.
- Hemicellulase...breaks down fiber .
- Lactase...breaks down milk sugar (is a type of carbohydrate) .

Fiber is known to help promote and maintains regularity, but most importantly, it helps to remove toxins, which are a major source of stress on the body. Fresh, unprocessed plant life contains fiber that stabilizes weight or aids in weight loss. Psyllium husk is also a good source of insoluble and soluble fiber.

Kelp is a seaweed, containing minerals, vitamins and trace elements. It, along with iodine content, affects the thyroid function, as well as other interactions with various drugs. It's important to verify, if it is appropriate.

Lactobacillus Acidophilus is a friendly bacteria when taking antibiotics. Unfortunately, antibiotics do not discriminate, as they kill both good and bad bacteria. Lactobacillus acidophilus helps strengthen and restore your body's internal balance. Here is a great tip: eat yogurt with active bacterial cultures to restore friendly bacteria. However, make sure to read the label to ensure it has the bacterial cultures!

Lecithin is a natural, occurring group of compounds found in every living cell and it coats the nerves. It is very important for brain function, such as memory and protects against cardiovascular disease, and provides cellular protection.

L-Tyrosine is an amino acid that aids in getting sleep.

Raw thymus and adrenal stimulate the functions of those glands, which are very helpful for dealing with stress in the body.

Proteolytic Enzymes destroy and release the free radicals that stress causes.

There are other supplementations and herbs that I prescribe, but as noted before, I tailor them according to my patient's specific needs and unique circumstances.

Diet

There is no one diet that is ideal for every cancer patient. All personal and individual needs must be taken into consideration. If not, the wrong diet, even if it is a perfectly healthy diet, may not be the answer to that person's cancer.

One should not expect even the best of diets to have any healing powers, if those healthy foods are ingested in a very toxic body environment and chemistry. Any poisons, drugs, chemicals or foreign substances present in the body fluids and tissues will immediately enter into a chemical reaction with those foods and contaminate, poison and de-nature them. They destroy our body's only biochemical healers – our enzymes.

The substances, which are originally foods, no longer have any ability to nourish or restore the body's needs.

Meals should be pleasant, relaxed and unhurried experiences; appetizing and appealing.

All meals must provide or contain a constant variety of plentiful quality oils: flax, sesame, sunflower and oil rich foods: seeds, grains, nuts in shells, avocados – every nutrient required for healing and health.

All foods in the diet must be: healthy and health restoring, fresh, full of their original life force and, as much as possible, organically grown; with no pesticides or chemical fertilizers, free from additives, preservatives, colorings or other chemicals. Well-salivated and chewed, eaten slowly and primarily vegetarian: vegetables, fruits, nuts, grains, seeds; a generous, but not excessive amount of quality proteins.

Special Precautions

- Always read labels before buying.
- Never buy anything that has ingredients you do not recognize as the food.
- Eat only when hungry.
- Do not eat if tired, exhausted, or hurried.

- Do not eat if angry, resentful, worried or upset.
- Do not eat when something is 'eating' you.
- Do not force foods or eat those you won't enjoy.
- Avoid over eating – eating beyond your hunger needs.

Special individual, nutritional needs would have to be determined by and analyzed for body chemistry, dietary habits and personality type. The most sophisticated systems for determining the latter is the computerized diagnostic system of healthEcel, Winthrop or Washington.

Holistic Healing

There many natural, powerfully effective ways to affect healing from cancer for our mind, body and spirit, and believe it or not, a lot of them are free of charge – graciously given to us by Mother Nature and divine power.

Exercising cannot be stressed enough, because it's healing qualities are quite profound, especially relieving the anxiety and depression that is often accompanied with cancer. Most people associate exercise with weight loss, but its value is worth far more than that. Even with cancer, there are many forms of exercise that are gentle, yet extremely beneficial: yoga, Tai Chi, Qi Gong are just a few that help in decreasing stress and increasing cardiovascular circulation, oxygenate the blood and cells, help the detoxification and elimination organs release toxins; strengthen the immune system, bring blood flow to the skin so that we are not looking gaunt and grey. It also strengthens memory and boosts energy. Having good energy makes us feel motivated, positive, confident, focused and relaxed.

Time and again, we've heard that the mind is the master of our healing. Our thoughts can be our adversary or our ally.

The practice of **visualizing** actually creates healing. We can direct our imagination to harmonize all the elements in our body into a peaceful state of optimal wellbeing and health restoration.

Meditation to calm the body and mind is also another healing practice, but most importantly, puts us in touch with our own divine power. For some people sitting quietly and stopping the mind's chatter is difficult. Listening to recordings of nature sounds or soft music can induce relaxed states. Or doing an activity that brings joy, such as gardening or playing a musical instrument where the mind completely focuses on it, is considered 'active' meditation.

We can reverse negative thoughts, habits, mindsets, emotions and disease. We have an inborn power to contribute to our recovery. Whatever occurs in our lives we can choose to use, to abuse or to reuse. The choice is ours. We can **affirm** by repeating...

"No one makes me angry, or creates guilt, fear, anxiety or worry in me. I do. I accept feelings of being worthless. I choose all my feelings. I choose hope and hopefulness. I am responsible for my choices. I must choose hope."

Today, some hospitals are using the healing and de-stressing power of **laughter** in their cancer departments. This idea is based on the work of Norman Cousins, author of *Anatomy of An Illness*, who was diagnosed with terminal cancer. His doctors' expectation was that he wouldn't live past many more months. He challenged their negative prognosis by using the power of the mind, combined with his body's natural wisdom to heal itself.

He isolated himself from the outside world, rented classic comedy films and laughed his way to wellness. Laughter, visualizing, plus nutritional supplements, primarily vitamin C and changes to his diet, cured his cancer. He lived decades beyond the doctors' prognosis. His last eight years of life were spent teaching at the world renowned Harvard Mind/Body Clinic in Boston, Massachusetts.

Talk therapy with a counselor or therapist to unburden and/or uncover what is hidden from our conscious awareness will help the healing process.

CHAPTER 7:
FINAL THOUGHTS

In all diseases there is purpose, positivity and blessings.
Dr. Leo Roy, MD, ND

I'd like to leave you with some guidelines and thoughts to ponder that are essential to your overall wellbeing.

In all diseases there is purpose, positivity and blessings. The manifestation of a disease are messages from the soul, demanding that we learn, change and eliminate all that is negative, hazardous and harmful in our lives, and to normalize our lifestyle. Diseases are warnings that tell us to never allow anything into our lives that could possibly be detrimental to our health.

Diseases can be a journey into the world of health – a first step on a joyful track to becoming one with life and with ourselves; an experience that could uncover greatness in our hearts and in us.

Dying in many ways is like the dying of a grain of wheat. Only in dying can a life, a beautiful plant, a beautiful flower and a beautiful fruit come into existence.

In a small village, at the foot of the Himalayas, lived a wise old man. His counsel was sought by people from miles around. A group of youngsters decided one day that they would make fun of this respected figure. They made a plan to expose his knowledge to ridicule. They would bring a bird, hidden behind the back of one of the boys. The boy would ask if the bird was alive or dead. If the old man said alive, the boy would crush it to death. If he said dead, the boy would release the bird. And so one day, the group approached the old man. One boy came forward to the village father and said,

"Father, what do I have in my hand?"

"A bird," he answered.

"Is the bird alive or dead?"

The old man looked up slowly and said gently, *"It is in YOUR hands".*

Your life, your healing, your happiness, your future wellbeing are in your hands. There are many things you, yourself personally can do to guarantee your success in overcoming cancer. You don't need a doctor for any of the following powerful healers. All you need is a little determination, willpower and perseverance.

Make up your mind to live – make it up to *really* live – to live it up – to enjoy and appreciate life to its fullest – to live *you* – the total you – your destiny and role on this earth – your purpose for living.

- Live one day at a time. Don't leave it until tomorrow.
- Live totally, mentally, physically, emotionally and socially.
- Listen to your soul and pray.
- Look to this day, for it is the life of your life.
- Take time to think, reflect and enjoy.
- Let go of the past.
- Do not anticipate the future.
- Live as intensely as you are able.
- Obtain the support of others.
- Do not let discouragement take over your mind.
- Avoid excesses, overloads, exhaustion.
- Release tensions by physical activities, exercise and enjoyments.
- Rest, relax and sleep a great deal.
- Adopt a health-restoring lifestyle.
- Believe curing is possible. Faith makes whole.
- Don't hurry. Don't worry.
- Keep joy in your life.

Don't give into temptation and go back to your old ways and excesses. It isn't worth it and stay away from spiteful, negative, irritating, overbearing people. You don't need friends who find fault with, and question your reasons for living your way to healing.

Deal promptly with discouragements, setbacks, lows, healing reactions.

If improvement is not felt in the early months of treatment, do not quit, give up or allow yourself to be discouraged. Discouragement and anxieties slow down healing.

Discomforts, reactions or changes in your condition should be constantly checked with your physician. Not doing so can lead to confusion, fears and healing failures.

Do not cease your treatment and health restoration for at least two years. To ease caring for your health and phasing out therapies your body needs before the healing process is complete, is leaving you wide open to a recurrence of your condition.

Detoxify, detoxify, detoxify! The tumor is not the real cancer.

The poisons and the deprivations we subject our body are the disease and the disease causes. Treat them.

And finally...

We are entering an age of enlightenment. We don't have to be chained to the ignorance of the past. We can look realistically at the hope for curing cancer in light of a great wealth of more recent research in the world of the living cells, our immune defense systems, and the role of our minds and emotions. We don't have to understand everything about our body's resisting abilities, but we can still use them. We don't understand electricity, yet we continue to use it.

Our bodies know more about how to cure and eliminate disease than science, chemistry and healing professions will ever know. What is understood can be corrected and managed, and very often cured.

Cancer is not incurable

- There is no incurable disease. There are masses of incurable people. There always will be.
- There is no cure for cancer. There never will be. There are only cures for people who have cancer.
- There is no universal system to cure cancer. There are only systems tailored specifically to the nature and needs of each individual patient.
- There is no simple, single therapy that can counteract multiple causes. Each cancer requires many systems and many remedies.
- There are common denominators and therapy needs for all cancer therapies: eliminating causes, detoxifying, correcting deficiencies and rebuilding host resistance.
- Cures exist only when all causes have been eliminated. Cures must be the total restoration of each body's need. Curing is balancing body chemistry, nervous system, hormones – all of

the body's needs. Curing is based on a reverence for life and reverence for nature.

- What is understood can be corrected and managed and very often cured.

Cancer does not mean that:

- You have to suffer.
- You have to die.
- You have to become a drug addict and a drug zombie.
- You have to be tortured by toxic, hazardous, painful, distressing treatments, the mutilation of surgery nor lethal chemotherapy or radiation.
- You have to lose your life's earnings on remedies, hospitals, and special care.
- You have to live in fear.

People who will remain incurable are those:

- Whose condition has passed beyond a stage of curability. They have ignored, neglected and allowed their condition to progress to a point of no return.
- Who do not want to, or will not accept curability.
- Who will not undertake the education, efforts and changes that can bring a cure into their body and life.
- Will not assume responsibility for their own health, happiness and health.
- Who prefer to believe that which has been believed over past centuries and persist in giving reference to science and chemistry rather than to nature and the nature of the life within them.
- Who have placed their bodies and their lives totally into the hands of another – even doctors – expecting them to do everything.
- Who do not have the means, the money, the help or the support they must have in order to overcome their disease.

REFEFRENCES

1. Wintergerst ES, Maggini S, Hornig DH. Immune-enhancing role of vitamin C and zinc and effect on clinical condition. Ann Nutr Metab 2006;50:85-94

2. Natural Health Products Directorate Monograph: Vitamin C. [Internet] [cited Oct 24th, 2007] Available at: http://www.hc-sc.gc.ca/dhp-mps/prodnatur/applications/licen-prod/monograph/mono_vitamin_c_e.html

3. Bagchi, C.K. Sen, M. Bagchi, and M. Atalay. Review: Anti-angiogenic, Antioxidant, and Anti-carcinogenic Properties of a Novel Anthocyanin-Rich Berry Extract Formula. [Internet] [cited on August 28/07]

4. Natural Medicines Comprehensive Database: Vitamin D. (Internet) (cited March 16, 2009):http://www.hc-sc.gc.ca/dhp-mps/prodnatur/applications/licen-prod/monograph/mono_vitamin_d-eng.php

5. *Mastery over Cancer: A Challenge to Live* [1998] by Dr. Leo Roy MD, ND

6. Magnesium: The Stress Reliever, Leo Galland, MD, FACN http://www.healthy.net/Health/Essay/Magnesium_The_Stress_Reliever/74 [Internet][cited, Sept. 7, 2015]

7. *Anatomy of an Illness* [1979] Norman Cousins, American political journalist, author, professor, and world peace advocate

8. *Scientific Roots of the Gerson Therapy* - Gehrardt Walker

ABOUT THE AUTHOR

Dr. Elvis Ali is highly respected for his work in Naturopathic Medicine. Dr. Elvis, as he is affectionately known, has been in private practice for almost 30 years, specializing in Chinese and sports medicine and nutrition. With impressive credentials - Bachelor of Science, majoring in Biology, Licensed Acupuncturist, Doctorate in Naturopathic Medicine; Mind/Body Medicine at Harvard Medical School, Diploma in Homeopathic Medicine - he lectures internationally, has written several books and appeared on radio and television shows. His passion lies in empowering people by educating them on complementary health and wellness and non-intrusive options.

Eat well, exercise and enjoy life.